PROSTAGLANDINS, PROSTACYCLIN, AND THROMBOXANES
MEASUREMENT

DEVELOPMENTS IN PHARMACOLOGY

VOLUME I

PROSTAGLANDINS, PROSTACYCLIN, AND THROMBOXANES MEASUREMENT

A Workshop Symposium on Prostaglandins, prostacyclin and thromboxanes measurement: methodological problems and clinical prospects, Nivelles, Belgium, November 15-16, 1979

Sponsored by the Commission of the European Communities, as advised by the Committee on Medical and Public Health Research

edited by

J.M. BOEYNAEMS
Department of Pharmacology
Vanderbilt University
Nashville, Tennessee, USA

and

A.G. HERMAN
Department of Pharmacology
University of Antwerp
Wilrijk, Belgium

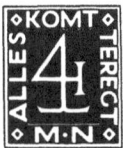

1980
MARTINUS NIJHOFF PUBLISHERS
THE HAGUE / BOSTON / LONDON

for

THE COMMISSION OF THE EUROPEAN COMMUNITIES

Distributors:

for the United States and Canada
Kluwer Boston, Inc.
190 Old Derby Street
Hingham, MA 02043
USA

for all other countries
Kluwer Academic Publishers Group
Distribution Center
P.O.Box 322
3300 AH Dordrecht
The Netherlands

for further information
Martinus Nijhoff Publishers by
P.O.Box 566
2501 CN The Hague
The Netherlands

ISBN-13: 978-94-009-8918-4   eISBN-13: 978-94-009-8916-0
DOI: 10.1007/978-94-009-8916-0

Publication arranged by:
Commission of the European Communities,
Directorate-General Scientific and Technical Information
and Information Management, Luxembourg

EUR 6859 EN

CONTENTS

CONTRIBUTORS

J.M. BOEYNAEMS
Department of Pharmacology
Vanderbilt University
Nashville, Tennessee, U.S.A.

A.R. BRASH
Division of Clinical Pharmacology
Vanderbilt University School of Medicine
Nashville, Tennessee, U.S.A.

F. CATTABENI
Institute of Pharmacology and Pharmacognosy
University of Milan
20129 Milan, Italy

M. CLAEYS
Faculty of Medicine
Division of Pharmacology
University of Antwerp
Universiteitsplein 1
B-2610 Wilrijk, Belgium

F. DRAY
FRA n°8 INSERM
Unité de Radioimmunologie Analytique
Institut Pasteur
28 rue Dr. Roux
75724 Paris Cedex 15, France

J.C. FROLICH
Dr.Margarete Fischer-Bosch-Institute
of Clinical Pharmacology
Auerbachstrasse 111
D-7000 Stuttgart 50, Germany

R.W. KELLY
Medical Research Council
Unit of Reproductive Biology
37 Chalmers Street
Edinburgh, Scotland

H. KINDAHL
Department of Obstetrics and Gynaecology
College of Veterinary Medicine
Swedish University of Agricultural Sciences
S-75007 Uppsala, Sweden

M. LAGARDE
Laboratoire d'Hémobiologie
Faculté Alexis Carrel
69372 Lyon Cedex 2, France

D.H. NUGTEREN
Unilever Research
P.O. Box 114
3130 AC Vlaardingen, The Netherlands

N.L. POYSER
Department of Pharmacology
1 George Square
Edinburgh, Scotland

J.A. SALMON
Department of Prostaglandin Research
Wellcome Research Laboratories
Langley Court
Beckenham
Kent BR 3 3 BS, England

F.A. FITZPATRICK
The Upjohn Company
Drug Metabolism Research
Kalamazoo, Michigan, U.S.A.

PREFACE

The rapid development in the knowledge about the synthesis and metabolism of the various products derived from arachidonic acid is a continuous challenge for those who intend to measure these substances in biological fluids. The confusion which still exists about their possible role in some physiological and pathological situations is partly due to the methodological problems related to the estimation of these metabolites in subnanogram quantities. This concern has inspired the Commission of the European Communities to sponsor a first workshop on the "Clinical Application of Assay Methods for Prostaglandins "which was held in Brussels at the end of 1976. During that meeting it became clear that progress in the qualitative and quantitative analysis of the prostaglandins could only be made by a permanent reevaluation of the existing techniques and therefore, the possibility should be created for experts in the field to meet regularly and to discuss the value of the newly developed assay methods.

Since then, exciting new discoveries have been made in this rapidly expanding area : in October 1976 the birth of the prostacyclin area was announced and in May 1979 a possible structure and biosynthetic pathway for slow-reacting substance of anaphylaxis (SRS-A) was presented. Since prostacyclin and thromboxane A_2 are very much involved in the platelet-vessel wall interaction, the measurement of these substances is a prerequisite in order to gain reliable information about their role in diseases such as atherosclerosis, arterial thrombosis, diabetic angiopathy, vasospasm, etc. This also applies for SRS-A (now called Leukotriene C or D), whose presence and activity during an asthmatic attack in humans has for long been hypothesized but has never been firmly established due to the lack of an assay method.

In view of the likely importance of the above mentioned substances, the Commission of the European Communities sponsored a second workshop on the methodological problems related to the estimation of some of the arachidonic acid methabolites. In accordance with the explicit wish of the Commission that the proceedings of that meeting should be quickly published the current volume contains the main contributions of that workshop including the highlights of the discussions which amply took place after each communication. Some chapters describe recent progress in the assay of 6-keto-PGF$_{1\alpha}$, the stable metabolite of prostacyclin, and of the products of the arachidonate lipxygenase, whereas others emphasize the potential pitfalls of these measurements and define criteria to establish their validity.

This book is not merely a collection of recipes, but it is the result of a meeting in which various experts had ample time and opportunity to discuss freely amongst each other the advantages and disadvantages of the existing or newly developed techniques. Furthermore, this meeting was not just another meeting in which everybody congratulated everybody on its recent achievements : on the contrary, due to the limited number of speakers and participants, no one hesitated to elaborate extensively on the possible drawbacks in the methods advocated by the others. Therefore we believe that this volume offers a valuable, original and up-to-date contribution to the advancement of our knowledge of the many facets of this intriguing group of antacoids which are called prostaglandins.

The Editors.

1 LIMITATIONS IN MEASUREMENT OF PROSTAGLANDINS AND THROMBOXANES

H. Kindahl and E. Granström

The development of quantitative methods, sensitive and specific enough for the measurement of the extremely small physiological amounts of prostaglandins and related compounds, has always constituted a great problem for researchers in the field. Published quantitative data display very wide discrepancies, even in studies of similar design. For example, reported "basal levels" of certain prostaglandins in peripheral plasma range from only 1 or 2 pg/ml to several ng/ml (1-6). Various sources of error probably contribute greatly to many of these results.

One common and serious mistake is the selection of an unsuitable compound for monitoring. As an example, in the past the primary prostaglandins were often measured in peripheral plasma samples, and measured concentrations were interpreted as the true endogenous levels. Most diverging results were obtained concerning the roles of these compounds in various conditions, such as for example pregnancy and labour (4, 7-9). Later it became clear that most of the measured amounts had been formed artifactually during the blood sampling. The artifactual production of prostaglandins in blood samples is likely to originate in platelets, white blood cells etc. Other biological fluids than blood may be free from this artifact. However, this must be ascertained before monitoring of the primary prostaglandins.

To avoid this confusing contribution in blood samples it is necessary to monitor the corresponding 15-keto-dihydro metabolites instead, which are not formed as artifacts,

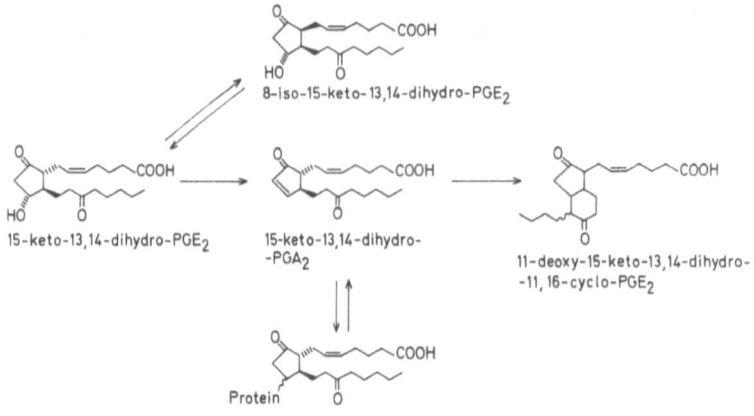

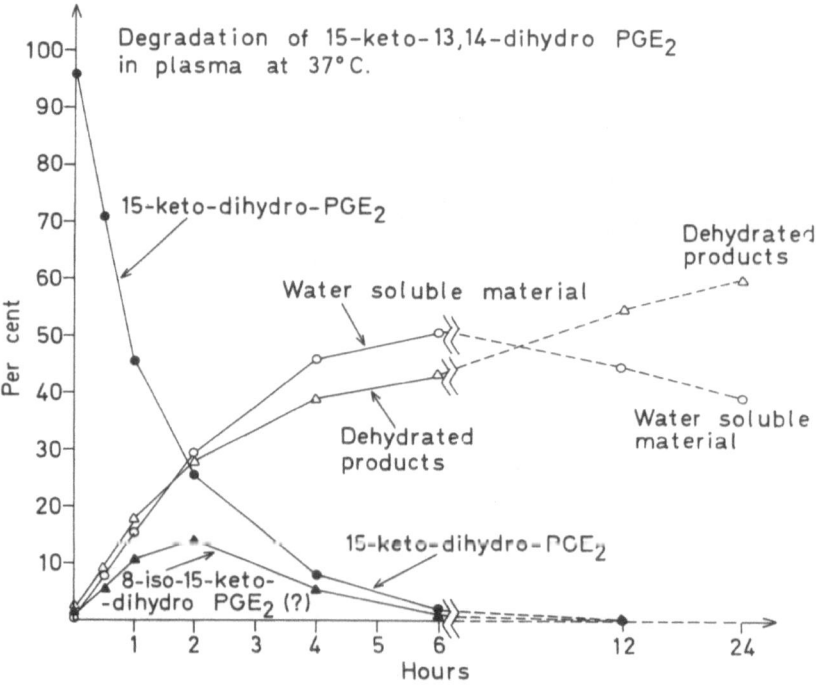

Fig. 1. Structures of products and tentative pathways in the degradation of 15-keto-13,14-dihydro-PGE₂ (upper panel), and the kinetics of degradation of ³H-15-keto-13,14-dihydro-PGE₂ in plasma at +37°C (lower panel).

which occur in higher amounts in the circulation, and which
have longer half-lives than the parent compounds (10,11).
This concept is now generally accepted and a large number
of studies has been performed where, for example, $PGF_{2\alpha}$ production has been followed during various biological events
by measurement of 15-keto-13,14-dihydro-$PGF_{2\alpha}$ as a reliable
indicator (11).

However, the situation has been far less bright for the
corresponding PGE_2 metabolite, 15-keto-13,14-dihydro-PGE_2.
Very few assays for this compound exist and consequently
very little is known about the biological roles of PGE_2.
Most scientists working with this metabolite have noticed
its pronounced instability. The fates of this compound were
recently elucidated (12,13): the compound is rapidly dehydra-
ted to 15-keto-dihydro-PGA_2 which is then cyclized to form
11-deoxy-13,14-dihydro-15-keto-11,16-cyclo-PGE_2 (Fig. 1,
upper panel). In plasma an additional fate is covalent binding to some plasma proteins such as albumin (Fig. 1, upper
panel). The kinetics of these events are illustrated in Fig.
1, lower panel, which indicates that all these reactions
must have occurred to a considerable extent during conditions
employed in several published assays for 15-keto-13,14-di-
hydro-PGE_2. The assay must then unintentionally have been
aimed at unknown and variable mixtures of all the degradation products. An obvious solution to the problem is to
monitor the final degradation product instead, the bicyclic
derivative, after this degradation has been induced to completion in all reagents and samples. This approach has recently been used in a radioimmunoassay (12).

In the thromboxane area the assay problems are even more
pronounced (Fig. 2). So far, no compound has been identified,
neither in the blood stream, nor in the urine which reliably
reflects thromboxane production in vivo and which thus would
be the obvious choice for monitoring (Fig. 2). When the
thromboxane pathway was discovered, it was first assumed
that the stable hydrolysis product, TXB_2, would be a good
indicator of TXA_2 synthesis, and several assays were deve-

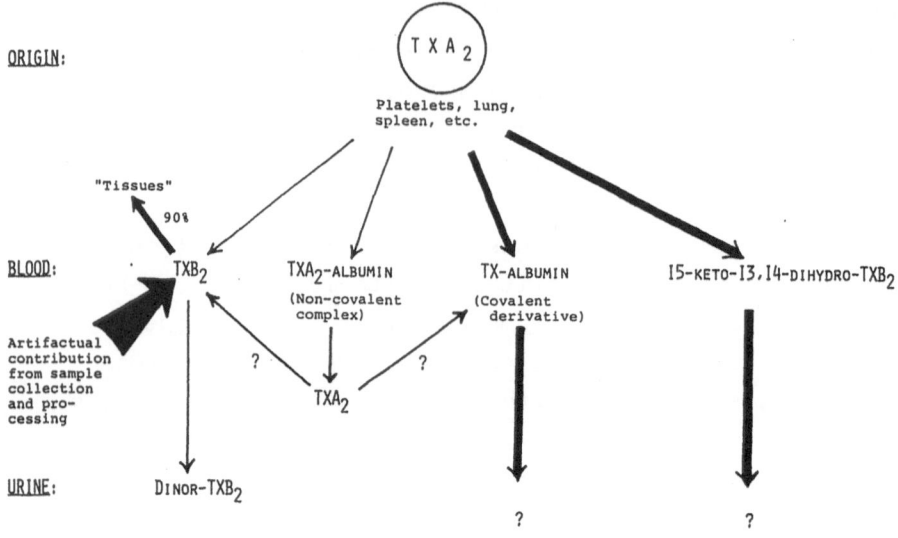

Fig. 2. Possible pathways in the metabolism of TXA_2. For
explanations, see text.

loped for this compound. This is probably the case in simpli-
fied biological systems, such as in washed platelets or in
subcellular fractions. In such systems it is even possible
to measure TXA_2, viz. as a derivative, mono-O-methyl-TXB_2,
formed directly from TXA_2 by treatment with excess of methanol (14). It is however unlikely that TXB_2 measurement in
for example plasma will be meaningful as an indicator of
thromboxane production in vivo. First, there is the same
problem with artifactual thromboxane synthesis by platelets
during the collection and handling of the sample as with the
primary prostaglandins, only much greater, as the thromboxane pathway is by far the dominating one in platelets. Second, in a study on the further fates of TXB_2 (15), it was
found that when TXB_2 was injected intravenously, about 90%
of the given dose was immediately taken up into tissues,

protein. Thus, the true events are reflected by the aliqouts
interrupted with acid. The same phenomenon was seen when
arachidonic acid was used to induce aggregation (24). Thus,
a major part of formed TXA_2 will be bound to albumin in
plasma and measurement of TXB_2 alone may lead to quite erro-
neous conclusions about the formation of thromboxanes.
Studies reporting low levels of TXB_2 in protein environments
should be reconciled in light of these recent findings.

Albumin binding of TXA_2 has been noticed earlier (25),
but in that study the opposite effect of albumin was studied,
viz. a non-covalent binding which exerted a protective effect
on the labile TXA_2 (Fig. 2). In neither case are the further
fates of the thromboxane derivatives known, such as the major, final urinary excretion products. Such knowledge would
probably solve the assay problems in the thromboxane field.

In addition to the metabolic and chemical problems so far
discussed, which are common to all assay methods, there are
several sources of error that particularly interfere with
radioimmunoassay.

A very important question in the field of radioimmunoassay is whether plasma samples must be extracted or if it
is possible to analyse unextracted samples. Prostaglandins
could be bound to albumin, like many other low molecular
weight substances (26). However, with the exception of the
covalent binding of thromboxanes and of α,β-unsaturated keto
compounds (such as PGA_2 or 15-keto-prostaglandins), the normal, non-covalent binding is weak and freely reversible (27).
In competition with antibodies of high avidity, the albumin
present in the sample should not interfere with the antibody
binding.

One reason for performing extraction is that it removes
undesirable substances that would interfere or cross-react
in the radioimmunoassay. Also in this respect the opposite
might rather hold true: in unextracted plasma the interfering substances could remain bound to albumin, in contrast
to the desired antigen, and are thus harmless, whereas extraction would strip the albumin molecules of many compounds

that may disturb the subsequent antigen-antibody binding. The most striking example of this is plasma fatty acids, which endogenously occur in plasma in concentrations around 200 µg/ml. In comparison, the levels of several prostaglandin metabolites are around 50 pg/ml or less. Although cross-reaction with straight chain fatty acids is always very low in prostaglandin or thromboxane assays, the high amounts present in the plasma would definitely interfere in the radioimmunoassay, if the fatty acids occurred free in the sample (28). Thus, unless the samples are not extensively purified after extraction to remove the fatty acids, a simple extraction procedure cannot be recommended. The possible influence of fatty acids in radioimmunoassay has recently been pointed out (29).

If extraction is deemed necessary for certain reasons, the extract must be further purified to remove the normal fatty acids and other compounds. However, many extraction, purification, and evaporation procedures unfortunately, seem to contribute further impurities to the final sample. One such example is shown in Fig. 3, which demonstrates the results from three different radioimmunoassays carried out on the eluate from a blank Amberlite XAD-2 column. The XAD-2 had been extensively washed before use, and the sample passed through the XAD-2 column was only 1 ml of redistilled water. From Fig. 3 it can be seen that very high amounts of interfering impurities are eluted with the methanol phase. These impurities are lipophilic degradation products from the resin, which evidently disturb the antigen-antibody binding. Many other procedures used for purification of prostaglandins, such as silicic acid chromatography and reversed phase partition chromatography, or even evaporation under a stream of nitrogen, may add further interfering impurities to the sample. When small biological samples have to be purified, and consequently whole fractions from chromatography columns have to be combined and evaporated to dryness before analysis, it is easy to understand that the results could be very erroneuos and not reflect any true biological events.

and, if redistrubuted into the blood stream, this process
was to slow to be measured. If this model mimics the situation after an endogenous release into the blood stream, detection of true endogenous TXB_2 levels becomes even more
difficult. Unfortunately no conversion of plasma TXB_2 into
15-keto-dihydro-TXB_2 has been noticed (15-17); otherwise
the occurrence of such a metabolite would have solved the
assay problem.

However, 15-keto-dihydro-TXB_2 has been identified as the
major product released after immunologic challenge of sensitized guinea pig lungs (18-20). It is thus possible that
endogenously formed thromboxane A_2 may be partially metabolized by different pathways than simply by hydrolysis into
TXB_2 (Fig. 2). A recent study of TXB_2 in vivo in sensitized
guinea pigs supports this assumption: after immunologic
challenge no increase was found in urine of the major degradation product of TXB_2, viz. dinor-TXB_2 (17). This indicates
how little information is provided by measurement of TXB_2
metabolites, since it is well known that TXA_2 is produced
in large amounts during anaphylaxis (21,22).

Also in in vitro experiments with platelets in plasma
misleading information about thromboxane production may be
obtained, when measuring TXB_2. In studies on the conversion
of PGH_2 into TXB_2 by platelet rich plasma, large differences
were noticed in measured TXB_2 levels when different methods
were used to interrupt the incubations (23). When acid was
added to the removed aliquots, measured TXB_2 levels indicated an intial burst of thromboxane production, followed by
a rapid disappearence. If acetone was used instead however,
no such burst was seen, but instead a slow continous increase in TXB_2 concentration was observed. This phenomenon
is explained by the fact that the formed TXA_2 is rapidly
trapped by plasma proteins, mainly albumin, forming covalently bound derivatives (24), and thus only a smaller part
of the formed TXA_2 is normally hydrolysed into TXB_2 (Fig. 2).
However, when the aliquots are treated with acid, the hydrolysis of TXA_2 into TXB_2 is more rapid than the binding to

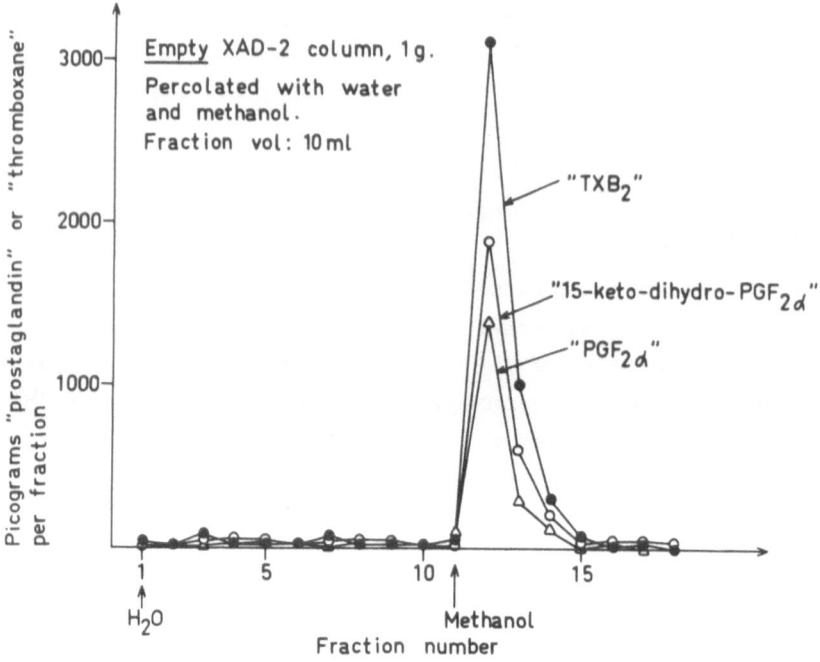

Fig. 3. Radioimmunoassay results obtained with three different assays on fractions from a chromatography of 1
ml of redistilled water on a column of Amberlite
XAD-2. Elution was carried out with water, followed
by methanol.

The identities of the majority of these disturbing factors
are not known. They are probably not chemically related to
prostaglandins or thromboxanes, and their interference in
radioimmunoassays is not simply caused by cross-reaction.
Instead the antigen-antibody binding is probably non-immuno-
logically inhibited by many of these substances. One compound which has caused a lot of problems in analytical work
is the ubiquitous impurity bis(2-ethyl-hexyl)phthalate ("di-

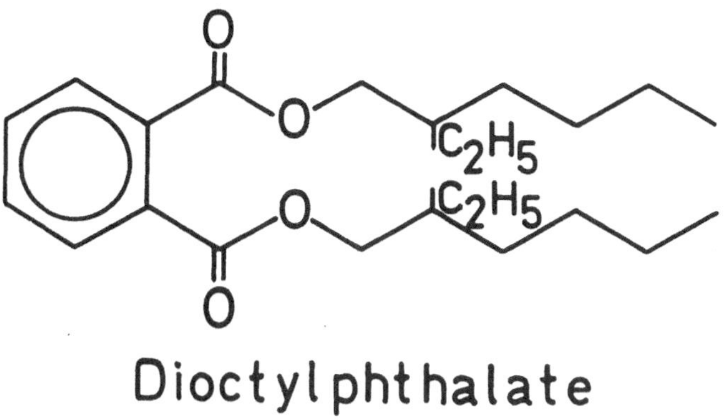

Dioctylphthalate

Fig. 4. Structure of bis(2-ethyl-hexyl)phthalate ("dioctyl-
      phthalate").

octylphthalate") (Fig. 4). This compound is a plasticizer,
present in oils, paints, all kinds of plastic utensils, etc
and has prostaglandin like properties in many chromatographic
systems. It has a slight structural resemblance with prostaglandins and thromboxanes, and since it may be present in
extremely high amounts in all "purified" samples, it might
also cause a true cross-reaction. Many scientists have noticed that the frequent use of plastic equipment in their
experimental procedure (tubes, catheters, pipette tips, etc)
inexplicably raises the "PG levels" in their samples. Procedure blanks can never compensate for all these disturbing
impurities, since true biological variations in the low
picogram range will be overshadowed by the variation in levels of impurities.

Since radioimmunoassay was introduced in the prostaglandir
field about 10 years ago many contradicting results have
been published using this method (e.g. the roles of prosta-

glandins in pregnancy and labour as already mentioned).
The explanation for the diverging results cannot be explained simply by differences in the properties of the different
antibodies employed, since they are often of good quality
(such as high avidity and high specificity). The large dis-
crepancies must instead be explained by differences in collection, storage, handling, and above all in processing of
the samples before radioimmunoassay as well as in the radioimmunoassay procedure itself. It must be emphasized that all
that radioimmunoassay does is to give information about the
degree of inhibition of the binding between the antibody and
the labelled ligand. Thus, one great problem with radioimmunoassay is that for a given sample, the method always results in a value, in contrast to many other assay methods.
The final radioactivity figure always falls somewhere on the
standard curve (unless very serious and specific sources of
error are involved). The obtained result must then be interpreted by the scientist: does it represent a true level, or
was it caused mainly by e.g. non-immunologic inhibition of
the binding? The situation is similar with computers: they
also provide an answer to a specific problem, which depends
on the information fed to the computer. An interesting expression has however emerged from this field, which also
may pertain to radioimmunoassay: "garbage in - garbage out"!

REFERENCES

1. Jaffe BM, Behrman HR, Parker CW: Radioimmunoassay measurement of prostaglandins E, A, and F in human plasma. J Clin Invest 52:398-405, 1973.

2. van Orden DE, Farley DB: Prostaglandin $F_{2\alpha}$ radioimmunoassay utilizing polyethylene glycol separation technique. Prostaglandins 4:215-233, 1973.

3. Zusman RM, Spector D, Caldwell BV, Speroff L, Schneider G, Mulrow PJ: The effect of chronic sodium loading and sodium restriction on plasma prostaglandin A, E and F concentrations in normal humans. J Clin Invest 52:1093-1098, 1973.

4. Hennam JF, Johnson DA, Newton JR, Collins WP: Radioimmunoassay of prostaglandin $F_{2\alpha}$ in peripheral venous plasma from men and women. Prostaglandins 5:531-542, 1974.

5. Youssefnejadian E, Walker E, Sommerville IF, Craft I: Simple direct radioimmunoassay of the F prostaglandins. Prostaglandins 6:23-35, 1974.

6. Dray F, Charbonnel B, Maclouf J: Radioimmunoassay of prostaglandins F_{α}, E_1 and E_2 in human plasma. Eur J Clin Invest 5:311-318, 1975.

7. Brummer HC: Serum $PGF_{2\alpha}$ levels during human pregnancy. Prostaglandins 3:3-5, 1973.

8. Gutierrez-Cernosek RM, Zuckerman J, Levine L: Prostaglandin $F_{2\alpha}$ levels in sera during human pregnancy. Prostaglandins 1:331-337, 1972.

9. Twomey SL, Bernett GE, Drewes PA: Serum prostaglandin $F_{2\alpha}$ levels during normal pregnancy. Clin Biochem 8:60-61, 1975.

10. Samuelsson B, Granström E, Gréen K, Hamberg M, Hammarström S: Prostaglandins. Ann Rev Biochem 44:669-695, 1975.

11. Samuelsson B, Goldyne M, Granström E, Hamberg M, Hammarström S, Malmsten C: Prostaglandins and thromboxanes. Ann Rev Biochem 47:997-1029, 1978.

12. Granström E, Kindahl H: Radioimmunologic determination of 15-keto-13,14-dihydro-PGE_2: A method for its stable degradation product, 11-deoxy-13,14-dihydro-15-keto-11β,16ξ-cycloprostaglandin E_2. In: Advances in Prostaglandin and Thromboxane Research, Vol. 6, Samuelsson B, Ramwell PW, Paoletti R (eds). Raven Press, New York, 1980, p. 181-182.

13. Granström E, Hamberg M, Hansson G, Kindahl H: Chemical instability of 15-keto-13,14-dihydro-PGE$_2$: The reason for low assay reliability. Prostaglandins, in press.

14. Granström E, Kindahl H, Samuelsson B: A method for measuring the unstable thromboxane A$_2$: Radioimmunoassay of the derived mono-0-methyl-thromboxane B$_2$. Prostaglandins 12:929-941, 1976.

15. Kindahl H: Metabolism of thromboxane B$_2$ in the cynomolgus monkey. Prostaglandins 13:619-629, 1977.

16. Roberts LJ, Sweetman BJ, Oates JA: Metabolism of thromboxane B$_2$ in the monkey. J Biol Chem 253:5305-5318, 1978.

17. Svensson J: Structure and quantitative determination of the major urinary metabolite of thromboxane B$_2$ in the guinea pig. Prostaglandins 17:351-365, 1979.

18. Dawson W, Boot JR, Cockerill AF, Wallen DNB, Osborne DJ: Release of novel prostaglandins and thromboxanes after immunological challenge of guinea pig lung. Nature 262: 699-702, 1976.

19. Boot JR, Cockerill AF, Dawson W, Mallen DNB, Osborne DJ: Modification of prostaglandin and thromboxane release by immunological sensitisation and successive immunological challenges from guinea-pig lung. Int Arch Allergy Appl Immunol 57:159-164, 1978.

20. Mallen DNB, Osborne DJ, Cockerill AF, Boot JR, Dawson W: Structural verification of 15-oxo-13,14-dihydrothromboxane B$_2$. Biomed Mass Spectrom 5:449-452, 1978.

21. Hamberg M, Samuelsson B: Prostaglandin endoperoxides VII. Novel transformations of arachidonic acid in guinea pig lung. Biochem Biophys Res Commun 61:942-949, 1974.

22. Piper PJ, Vane JR: Release of additional factors in anaphylaxis and its antagonism by anti-inflammatory drugs. Nature 223:29-35, 1969.

23. Fitzpatrick FA, Gorman RR: Platelet rich plasma transforms exogenous prostaglandin endoperoxide H$_2$ into thromboxane A$_2$. Prostaglandins 14:881-889, 1977.

24. Maclouf J, Kindahl H, Granström E, Samuelsson B: Thromboxane A$_2$ and prostaglandin endoperoxide H$_2$ form covalently linked derivatives with human serum albumin. In: Advances in Prostaglandin and Thromboxane Research, Vol. 6, Samuelsson B, Ramwell PW, Paoletti R (eds). Raven Press, New York, 1980, p. 283-286.

25. Folco G, Granström E, Kindahl H: Albumin stabilizes thromboxane A$_2$. FEBS Lett 82:321-324, 1977.

26. Spector AA: Fatty acid binding to plasma albumin. J Lipid Res 16:165-179, 1975.

27. Unger WG: Binding of prostaglandin to human serum albu-
    min. J Pharm Pharmacol 24:470-477, 1972.

28. Gold EW, Edgar PR: The effect of physiological levels of
    nonesterified fatty acids on the radioimmunoassay of
    prostaglandins. Prostaglandins 16:945-952, 1978.

29. Metz S, Rice M, Robertson RP: Applications and limita-
    tions of measurement of 15-keto,13,14-dihydro prosta-
    glandin E_2 in human blood by radioimmunoassay. Prosta-
    glandins 17:839-861, 1979.

DISCUSSION

A. Brash   I would like to make two comments about the calculation
                made on the predicted levels of $PGF_{2\alpha}$ in peripheral
                plasma (Reference : Samuelsson – Adv.Biosciences 9.)
                Firstly the levels measured during infusion of $PGF_{2\alpha}$
                (200 μg/min) were performed using pregnant women and
                there is evidence from animal studies that the levels of
                15 – OH dehydrogenase are elevated during pregnancy.
                Thus more metabolite and comparatively less $PGF_{2\alpha}$ may
                have been found than if non-pregnant subjects were
                studied. Secondly it is obvious that intravenous infusion
                of $PGF_{2\alpha}$ does not mimic in vivo production in tissues.
                We must remember that these predicted levels of $PGF_{2\alpha}$
                in peripheral plasma are indeed just calculations.

N. Poyser   Cross-reactivities alone may be misleading since the fatty
                acids, although present in large quantities, may have low
                affinity for the antibody and will be displaced by low
                quantities of the prostaglandin which has high affinity
                for the antibody.

H. Kindahl   I agree with you and the best way to check the true in-
                fluence of the fatty acids should be to combine different
                amounts of the fatty acid under study with the prostaglandin
                which the RIA is developed for. But still the very high
                amounts of fatty acids could disturb your results. I believe
                that albumine helps you in this respect and binds a lot of
                the fatty acids, thus the influence of the fatty acids
                becomes less important.

F.A. Fitzpatrick   The 11-deoxy-11,16 bicyclo-dihydro-15 keto-PGE_2
contains at least two centers of assymetry
Is it epimerically pure after base treatment?
I bring this up because some samples I examined by
HPLC, supplied by Upjohn, contain at least two epimers
of approximately equal concentration?

H. Kindahl   The bicyclic compound appears as three peaks on HPLC
and the fourth possible epimer might cochromatograph with
one of the **epimers**.

P. Lijnen   1. Does 13, 14-dihydro-15 Keto-PGE_2 degrade also at
0 - + 2°C, e.g. when the blood samples are with-
drawn into chilled tubes and centrifuged immediately
to remove the platelets?
2. Can you solve the instability of the standard in the
radioimmunoassay by using ethanol instead of buffer?
3. Does this metabolite change during prolonged
storage of plasma in the freezer at -20°C ?
4. Is it possible to exclude protein-binding of this
metabolite by extraction of the plasma samples with
organic solvents ?

H. Kindahl   1. The platelets are not important for the dehydration.
The dehydration slows down in the chilled samples
but you cann't stop it. The same is true for storage
of plasma at -20°C.

2. The stability is better in ethanol, but you always
have the problem of dehydration in the condition
for the RIA-incubation.

3. Of course you can decrease the importance of protein
binding by extracting your samples, however the
dehydration continues.

F.Cattabeni   You mentioned that with XAD_2 column you get out
material which cross reacts in the RIA. Have you any
idea whether these interfering compound could interfere also with the mass fragmentographic assay?

H. Kindahl   I am absolutely sure that this is the case, and that very
extensive further purification of the samples is needed.

R.Kelly   (in context of binding of endoperoxides, thromboxane A_2 to
protein)
Have you any idea of the groups within the protein
molecule to which you expect the endoperoxides and
thromboxane to bind?

H. Kindahl   We don't know which groups are involved in this binding; it might be the same groups for both endoperoxides
and TXA_2

J. Salmon   If I may break away from methodology for a moment.
There have been reports that thromboxane B_2 is elevated
in patients with angina. Do you have any experience
with measuring TXB_2 in pathological conditions.

H. Kindahl   I have never studied thromboxane production in vivo,
since today no good methods exist. TXB_2 or TXB_2-meta-
bolites (e.g. dinor-TXB_2) reflects very badly TXA_2
production in vivo. Instead I have studied some pathological platelet conditions in vitro and measured
thromboxane production after different stimuli.

2 SENSITIVITY AND SPECIFICITY OF PROSTANOIC DERIVATIVES RADIOIMMUNOASSAYS: NEW APPROACH

F. Dray

Prostanoic derivatives, as prostaglandin, thromboxane, prostacyclin and their metabolites, are generally present in biological media at very low concentrations (10^{-9} - 10^{-11}M). Therefore assays with high sensitivity often are required for their measurement. Two techniques are widely used : mass spectrometry combined with gas chromatography (GS-MS), which is particularly specific (1) and radio-immunoassay (RIA) which particularly sensitive and convenient for large series (2,7). In our laboratory, immuno-logical methods have been developed using radioactive (8) or non-radioactive tracers (5,9); iodinated derivatives (as PG-^{125}I-Histamine) have been shown to be more sensitive and convenient (10-14). In this paper some aspects of the use of iodinated tracers will be presented and a new approach for increasing the specificity of prostanoic derivatives will be proposed.

PREPARATION AND SELECTION OF IMMUNE SERA.

Preparation of the immunogen

To act as immunogens, PGs are covalently linked to an antigenic carrier. The chemical action selected must enable an adequate number of molecules to be bound to the carrier, and maintain the structural integrity of the molecule (except for the group involved in the covalent bond with the antigenic carrier). In our experiments, we used bovine serum albumin (BSA) as the carrier; the free carboxyl function of the hapten, activated by a carbodi-imide, forms a peptide bond with the free NH_2 groups of the antigenic carrier (8). Under our conditions (shown

in table I) in most experiments 15 to 20 moles of PG
were bound per mole BSA.

Immunisation

Animals were administered the PG-BSA conjugate according to a method originally proposed by Vaitukaitis et
al. (15). Each rabbit received 30-40 intradermal injections of the conjugate (about 200 µg) dissolved in 1 ml
physiological buffered saline and emulsified in an equal
volume of Freund's complete adjuvant. Five animals were
immunised in each series.

Booster injections, given two months after the primary
injections, were carried out following the same schedule.
Subsequent booster injections were given depending upon
the development of antibody titre. These subsequent
booster injections, using smaller amounts of antigen,
were carried out when the antibody titre fell from a
maximum value. Animals were bled every ten days after
the fourth week of immunisation.

Study of binding parameters

The course of the immune response may be followed by
measuring the titre of the antiserum, defined as the
dilution giving 50% binding of the radioactive tracer.
When the titre of the serum was high enough, its sensitivity, affinity and specificity were tested. The best
bleedings were kept separately or pooled. They were
stored either at +4°C after addition of 0.02% sodium
azide, or at -20°C after dilution in an equal volume of
glycerol. Table 2 shows the specificity of certain selected antisera.

Table I. Preparation of prostaglandin immunogen

	REAGENT	QUANTITY (mg)	VOLUME (ml)	MEDIUM	REACTION TIME
STEP 1 (COOH ACTIVATION)	PG + (^{3}H)-PG	10	10	Sodium carbonate	
	+				
	E D C I*	10		pH 5.5	1 h.
STEP 2 (COUPLING)	+			Sodium carbonate	
	BOVINE SERUM ALBUMIN	20	10	pH 5.5	Overnight

*1-Ethyl-3 (3-dimethyl-amino-propyl)-carbodiimide-HCl

- All reactions are carried out at room temperature

- Conjugate is dialysed against distilled water for 24 h. at +4°C

- Number of PG-residues per molecule of albumin is estimated on the basis of isotopic dilution.

Table 2. Specificity of some prostaglandin derivatives antisera.

ANTISERUM	INHIBITORS									
	E_1	E_2	$F_{1\alpha}$	$F_{2\alpha}$	DHK E_2	DHK $F_{2\alpha}$	TXB_2	$6\text{-}K\text{-}F_{1\alpha}$	$19\text{-}OH\text{-}F_{2\alpha}$	$19\text{-}OH\text{-}E_2$
E_1	100	~5	0.2	<0.1	–	<0.1	–	–	–	–
E_2	3	100	<0.1	0.1	0.1	<0.1	–	–	–	–
$F_{1\alpha}$	0.1	<0.1	100	7	<0.1	<0.1	–	–	<0.1	<0.1
$F_{2\alpha}$	0.3	0.8	29	100	<0.1	4	–	–	<0.1	<0.1
DHK E_2	<0.5	<0.5	<0.5	<0.5	100	7	–	–	–	–
DHK $F_{2\alpha}$	<0.1	<0.1	<0.1	<0.1	<0.1	100	–	–	–	–
TXB_2	<0.1	<0.1	–	<0.1	<0.1	<0.1	100	–	<0.1	<0.1
$6\text{-}K\text{-}F_{1\alpha}$	6	2	18	11	–	0.3	<0.1	100	0.2	<0.1
$19\text{-}OH\text{-}F_{2\alpha}$	–	–	4	2	–	–	–	–	100	<0.1
$19\text{-}OH\text{-}E_2$	35	23	–	0.2	–	–	–	–	–	100

Cross reactivities are calculated on the basis of quantity (pg) necessary for 50% tritiated tracer displacement.

20

PREPARATION OF IODINATED TRACERS

Preparation of PG derivatives

A PG "derivative" was synthesised as the substrate for iodination. For our studies the PG molecule was coupled to histamine; in preliminary work tyramine or tyrosyl methyl ester was used and similar binding parameters were obtained (10). A peptide bound was formed between the free NH_2 group of histamine and the free COOH group of PG (Table 3); the derivative then was purified and separated from the reagents by thin layer chromatography on silica gel in n-butanol/acetic acid/water system (75:10:25 v/v). The addition of (^{3}H)-histamine to the reaction mixture in a preliminary experiment allowed localization and identification the derivative formed (fig. 1). After elution in methanol, the derivative was distributed in small fractions and lyophilized.

Iodination procedure

The method of Hunter and Greenwood (16) with chloramine T was used to incorporate ^{125}iodide in the imidazol ring of histamine. Table 4 and Fig. 2 show the iodination procedure and the distribution of the radioactivity after purification on thin layer chromatography of the 6,15-diketo-PGF$_{1\alpha}$, which is a metabolite of prostacyclin.

Table 3. Preparation of prostaglandin-histamine derivative

	REAGENT	QUANTITY (μmol)	VOLUME (ml)	MEDIUM	REACTION TIME
STEP 1 (COOH ACTIVATION)	PG + E D C I*	28.6 52	0.5	Ethanol-water 1:1, v/v	1 h.
STEP 2 (COUPLING)	+ HISTAMINE (His)	90	0.5	Water	Overnight

*1-Ethyl-3 (3-dimethyl-amino-propyl)-carbodiimide-HCl

- All reactions are carried out at room temperature.

Table 4. Iodination procedure

PRODUCT	VOLUME (μl)	CONCENTRATION AND BUFFER
PG-His	10	$\approx$ 1 nmol.
Phosphate buffer	10	0.5M, pH 7.4
Na^{125}I	2	100 Ci/ml
Chloramine T	2	2.5 mg/ml in phosphate buffer

- 20 seconds reaction time; stopped with sodium metabi-sulfite (32 μg)
- (^{125}I)-PG-His is purified by TLC (silica gel) in chloroform/water (60:30:5, v/v).
- Radioactive spot is located by autoradiography and iodinated product is eluted from silica gel by ethanol and stored after distribution into small fractions at -20°C until use.

THE RADIOIMMUNOLOGICAL REACTION

The method varies depending upon whether an iodinated or a tritiated tracer is used.

RIA using a tritiated tracer

To 5 ml polystyrene tubes were added successively 0.1 ml tritiated tracer (about 7,500 dpm), 0.1 ml PG standard or biological extract and 0.1 ml of a dilution of the antiserum such that the initial binding in the absence of standard or unknown PG is 40-50% of the total radioactivity. All the reagents were diluted in phosphate-buffered saline at pH 7.4, 0.1M, 0.9% NaCl, 0.1% gelatin. The tubes were incubated overnight at 4°C. Separation of the free fraction from that bound to the antiserum was carried out at 0°C by the addition of 1 ml charcoal-dextran. After incubation for 12 minutes in a melting ice bath, the tubes were centrifuged for 15 min. at 2000 g. The supernatant (bound fraction) was transferred to scintillation vials and counted in a liquid

scintillation counter for 4 minutes. The standard curve
was determined by plotting the log of the dose (pg/tube)
on the abscissa against the value (%) of the ratio B/Bo
(B being the amount of radioactivity bound to the antibody)on the ordinate. The results were then calculated
by computer.

RIA using iodinated tracers

   The technique is basically the same as for tritiated
tracers, with the following modifications : 14,000 dpm
iodinated tracer was added to each tube, and the buffer
used contained 0.3% bovine gamma globulin instead of
gelatin. Free and bound radioactivity were separated by
adding 0.3 ml polyethylene glycol 6000 at 0°C to each
tube (25 g/100 ml distilled water), mixing well and centrifuging at +4°C for 15 minutes at 2000 g. The supernatant was decanted and the pellet (the bound fraction) was
counted for 1 minute in a gamma counter.

Binding parameters of RIAs using iodinated tracers

   These were tested for each antiserum in comparison
with tritiated tracer. We always observed a higher
dilution of the antiserum to bind 50% of tracer, usually
no significant alteration of percentage of cross-reac-
tions and very often an increase in sensitivity. This
last point will be discussed later.

PURIFICATION OF BIOLOGICAL SAMPLES

   Sampling of biological fluids (blood, urine, amniotic fluid, etc ...) or tissues should be carried out according to a standard procedure adapted for each biological medium. Biosynthesis and metabolism of prostaglandins in the sample must be inhibited. In the case of urine, for example, each miction was collected in a clean vessel and immediately transferred to a bottle at 4°C containing meclofenamic acid. The total volume was measured after 24 hours and a fraction stored at -20°C.

Extraction

   Two ml urine sample was pipetted into a centrifuge tube containing about 1800 dpm of appropriate ^{3}H tracer for calculation of the extraction recovery. After acidification to pH 3.5 with citric acid, the PGs were extracted from the sample with three volumes of a mixture of cyclohexane and ethyl acetate (1:1, v/v). After 15 min. vigorous shaking and centrifugation at 250 g, the organic phase was pipetted into a conical siliconised tube. The extraction was repeated and the two extracts pooled and evaporated to dryness under nitrogen.

CHROMATOGRAPHIC PURIFICATION

- ### Silicic acid chromatography

Prostanoic derivatives were purified by passage
over a silicic acid column : 500 mg silicic acid was
equilibrated in 2 ml solvent 2 and washed first with
5 ml benzene/ethyl acetate/methanol (60:40:20, v/v)
solvent 3), and then with 1.5 ml solvent 2. The
extract was re-dissolved in 0.2 ml benzene/ethyl ace-
tate/methanol (60:40:20, v/v) (solvent 1) and 0.5 ml
benzene/ethyl acetate (60:40, v/v) (solvent 2), the
total volume of the extract was placed on the column
and the compounds were eluted by three successive
solvents :

. Elution 1 : 6 ml solvent 2 to extract the less polar
  lipids, pigments, PGA, PGB and 13,14-dihydro-15-Keto-
  PGE_1 or PGE_2

. Elution 2 : 13 ml solvent 4 (benzene/ethyl acetate/
  methanol, 60:40:2, v/v) to extract PGE_1 and PGE_2
  and also 13,14-dihydro-15-Keto-$PGF_{1\alpha}$ and $F_{2\alpha}$

. Elution 3 : 4 ml solvent 3 to extract PGs F_α and
  19-OH-PGE and F_α

Each eluate was evaporated under nitrogen and redissolved in an adequate quantity of buffer for radioimmunological assay. A portion was used to calculate recovery for the extraction and purification processes.

When thromboxane B_2, 6-keto-PGF$_{1\alpha}$ and 6,15-diketo-
$PGF_{1\alpha}$ have to be measured elutions 2 and 3 were replaced
by only one elution with 5 ml solvent 2.

High performance liquid chromatography (HPLC)

The eluate after silicic acid column was evaporated
to dryness, then injected onto a column of µBondapack C_{18}
(Waters) with elution conditions allowing the best separation of PGs and related compounds (Fig. 3). The content
of tubes was evapored and RIA was carried out on each.

COMMENT

PROBLEMS ARISING FROM THE USE OF IODINATED TRACERS
PREPARED FROM PG-HISTAMINE DERIVATIVES.

Use of an iodinated derivative as a pose to a tritiated tracer modifies, to a greater or lesser extent, the
competitive properties of the immunological system invol-
ved.There are two main factors involved:

The specific activity of the iodinated tracer

The specific activity of the iodinated tracer is
considerably higher than that of a tritiated tracer,
and, with appropriate purification, may be as high as
that of sodium iodide (about 2000 Ci/mmole). In such
cases, the weight of the tracer becomes very small and
is no longer a limiting factor in the sensitivity of
the assay.

The structure of the iodinated derivative

The COOH function of the prostaglandin molecule is
blocked in the formation of the peptide bridge. This
increases its similarity of structure to the immunogen.
Certain populations of antibodies, however, may selecti-
vely recognise the peptide bridge region of the molecule
and recognise less, or not at all,the prostaglandin part
of the iodinated tracer. In all situations where there
is a difference in the structures of the ligand and the
radioactive tracer, the thermoaynamic properties of the
competitive system will be modified.

This system, it should be remembered, involves the isotopic dilution of a reaction which obeys the law of mass action, according to the equation :

$$Ag^* + Ac + Ag \rightleftharpoons Ag^* - Ac + Ag - Ac$$

$$
\begin{aligned}
&Ag^* \quad \text{tracer} \quad \text{unbound} \\
&Ag \quad \text{ligand unbound} \\
&Ac \quad \text{antibody unbound}
\end{aligned}
$$

and at equilibrium :

$$Ka^* = \frac{Ag^* - Ac}{Ag^* \quad Ac} \quad \text{and} \quad Ka = \frac{Ag - Ac}{Ag - Ac}$$

Ka^* and Ka = association constant for each competitor expressed in L/M

In the case of a tritiated tracer, where there is homology between the structure of the ligand and the tracer, equations are identical and $Ka^* = Ka$

Where in the case of an iodinated tracer, theoretically there are three possible results.

1) $^*Ka < Ka$: there is marked heterology of the two competitors (existence of a bridge, presence of iodine) and the iodinated tracer is not so whell recognised by the antibody binding sites as is the unlabelled prostaglandin. In limiting cases the iodinated tracer not participate in the competition.

2) $^*Ka > Ka$: The structure of the iodinated derivative resembles that of the immunogen more closely than that of the competitor, and may, in extreme cases, be so different from the competitor that it cannot be displaced. The competitive system can only function if the Ka can be elevated by modifying the structure of the ligand. Table 5 shows that the sensitivity is often improved when the carboxyl group of the ligand is esterified as methyl ester (13).

3) $^*Ka \neq Ka$: In this, the best situation, the radioactivity is higher, the dilution of the antiserum is greater and the competitive system functions well at lower concentrations of ligand, which diminishes the detection threshold (Table 6). In addition, the cross reactions are only slightly modified when compared with the homologous system using tritiated tracer.

PROBLEMS CONCERNING THE VALIDITY OF PROSTAGLANDIN RADIOIMMUNOASSAY

These problems are threefold :

1) The radioimmunoassay system itself, in which can be distinguished permanent factors : the parameters of antibody binding (affinity, specificity), the relative affinity of the competitors for the antibody sites, and the experimental conditions and separation of bound and free, and contingent factors related to individual assays, material present in the biological fluids or introduced or concentrated during the purification procedures.

2) The purification of samples prior to radioimmunoassay; the extent of the purification depends on the circonstances : in the case of a new prostanoic derivative or a new biological milieu, we systematically employ all the steps shown in the fig. 4.

The assay of 6-Keto-PGF$_{1\alpha}$ in urine is an example of the necessity of carrying out all these procedures (Table 7). In other cases, however, experience has shown that one or more of the steps may be omitted, and in some cases, a direct assay of the solution of biological sample may be carried out. In these cases, the results obtained after omission of each step must be compared, to ensure that simplification does not engender error. For instance, it has now been shown that for PGE and PGF$_\alpha$ assay, a purification using HPLC is not necessary, that often, with our antisera, the results obtained in

the assay of PGE_2 after a simple extraction procedure
are valid; that TXB_2 may be assayed directly in a diluted
biological sample such as serum.

3) The sampling technique. For bioassay, GC/MS and RIA,
rigorous and reproducible conditions of sampling, and
subsequent treatment of samples, must be established.
These should be adapted to each individual biological
medium so as to reduce to a minimum the in vitro transformation by synthesis or degradation, of the prostanoic
derivatives analysed.

In this way, the quantitative analysis of these
compounds is of value and may be an invaluable tool
for the research biologist and also the clinician.

Table 5. Sensitivities of prostaglandins antisera using tritiated and iodinated tracers.

TRACER	ANTISERA							
	E_1	E_2	$F_{1\alpha}$	$F_{2\alpha}$	DHK E_2	DHK $F_{2\alpha}$	TXB_2	$6\text{-}K\text{-}F_{1\alpha}$
(^3H)-PG [a]								
SENSITIVITY [a]	32	5	15	3.5	54	8	14	94
SPECIFIC RADIOACTIVITY (Ci/mmol)	90	117	79	178	66	85	125	20
FINAL DILUTION OF ANTISERUM	1/45,000	1/75,000	1/15,000	1/90,000	1/3,600	1/45,000	1/24,000	1/13,500
(^{125}I)-PG-His [b]								
SENSITIVITY	18	2.5	29	7	33	5	8	15
FINAL DILUTION	1/300,000	1/150,000	1/25,000	1/105,000	1/15,000	1/150,000	1/45,000	1/168,000

[a] Quantity of PG (pg) necessary to give 50% displacement of Bo : for all assays, the final dilution of the antiserum was adjusted to obtain 50-40% initial binding.

[b] Specific radioactivity of (^{125}I)-labelled PG-histamine tracers was estimated to 2000 Ci/mmol.

Table 6. Concentration of PG required (pmol/ml) to give 50% displacement of Bo using different tracers and inhibition.

TRACER/INHIBITOR	SYSTEM					
	PGE_1	PGE_2	$PGF_{1\alpha}$	$PGF_{2\alpha}$	DHK PGE_2	DHK $PGF_{2\alpha}$
(^{125}I)-labeled-PG-His/PG	0.17	0.025	0.82	0.20	0.95	0.09
(^{125}I)-labeled-PG-His/PG-ME [a]	0.09	0.028	0.14	0.08	0.26	0.09

[a] Abbreviation : ME, methyl ester

Table 7. Urinary 6-Keto-PGF$_{1\alpha}$ of 3 healtly adult women (pg/ml)

RIA after	1	2	3
a) Silicic acid column	2974	5003	3085
b) HPLC*			
. Immunoreactivity of all the fractions	657	1937	1157
. Immunoreactivity of the peak correspon- ding only to 6-Keto-PGF$_{1\alpha}$ standard	284	620	313

*See the profile of fig. 3 A.

REFERENCES

1. Green, K. Advanc. Biosci. $\underline{9}$, 91-108 (1973)

2. Levine, L. and Van Vanukis, H. Biochem. Biophys.
   Res. Commun. $\underline{41}$, 1171-1177 (1970)

3. Cadwell, B.V., Burstein, S., Brock, W.A. and
   Speroff, L. J. Clin. Endocr. Metab. $\underline{33}$, 171-175
   (1971)

4. Jaffe, B.M., Smith, J.W., Newton, W.T. and Parker,
   C.W. Science, $\underline{171}$, 494-496 (1971)

5. Dray, F., Maron, E., Tillson, S.A. and Sela, M.
   Anal. Biochem. $\underline{50}$, 399-408 (1972)

6. Kirton, K.T., Cornette, J.C. and Barre, K.L.
   Biochem. Biophys. Res. Commun. $\underline{47}$, 903-909 (1972)

7. Dray, F. and Charbonnel, B. Colloque INSERM 1973
   pp. 133-158

8. Dray, F., Charbonnel, B. and Maclouf, J. Europ.
   J. Clin. Invest. $\underline{5}$, 311-318 (1975)

9. Andrieu, J.M., Mamas, S. and Dray, F. Prostaglandins, $\underline{6}$, 15-22 (1974)

10. Maclouf, J., Pradel, M., Pradelles, P. and Dray, F.
    Biochem. Biophys. Acta, $\underline{431}$, 139-146(1976)

11. Sors, H., Maclouf, J., Pradelles, P. and Dray, F.
    Biochem. Biophys. Acta, $\underline{486}$, 553-564 (1977)

12. Sors, H., Pradelles, P., Dray, F., Rigaud, M.,
    Maclouf, J. and Bernard, P. Prostaglandins, $\underline{16}$,
    277-290 (1978)

13. Maclouf, J., Sors, H., Pradelles, P. and Dray, F.
    Anal. Biochem. $\underline{87}$, 169-176 (1978)

14. Dray, F., Gerozissis, K., Kouznetzova, B., Mamas, S.,
    Pradelles, P. and Trugnan, G. Advances in prosta-
    glandin and Thromboxane Research, Vol. 6, edited by
    B.Samuelsson, P.W.Ramwell and R.Paoletti. Raven
    Press, N.Y. (1980) pp. 167-180

15. Vaitukaitis, J., Robbins, J.B., Nieschlag, E. and
    Ross, T. J. Clin. Endocr. $\underline{33}$, 988-990 (1971)

16. Hunter, W.N. and Greenwood, F.C. Nature, $\underline{194}$,
    495-496 (1962)

LEGENDS FIGURES

Fig. 1 : Thin-layer chromatography on silica gel for the purification of 6,15-diketo-PGF$_{1\alpha}$ coupled to histamine.(see the text for details)

Fig. 2 : Thin-layer chromatography on silica gel : distribution of the radioactivity (see the text for details).

Fig. 3 : Separation of various prostaglandins and metabolites by HPLC. Application to analyse the 6-Keto-PGF$_{1\alpha}$ (3 A), PGF$_{2\alpha}$ (3 B) and PGE$_2$ (3 C) immunoreactive component in human urine ( ).

Conditions = Instrument : Waters Associates
            Packing   : μBondapack C$_{18}$
            Column   : 3.9 mm x 30 cm
            Flow rate : 1 ml/min.
            Solvent   : A = acetonitrile/water
                             (5:95, v/v)
                         B = acetonitrile/water
                             (95:5, v/v)

Model 660 solvent programmer for 1 h. curve 8. Starting solvent 17% B in A - final solvent 100% B.

Fig. 4 : Schema proposed for purification of extracts before "PG" RIA

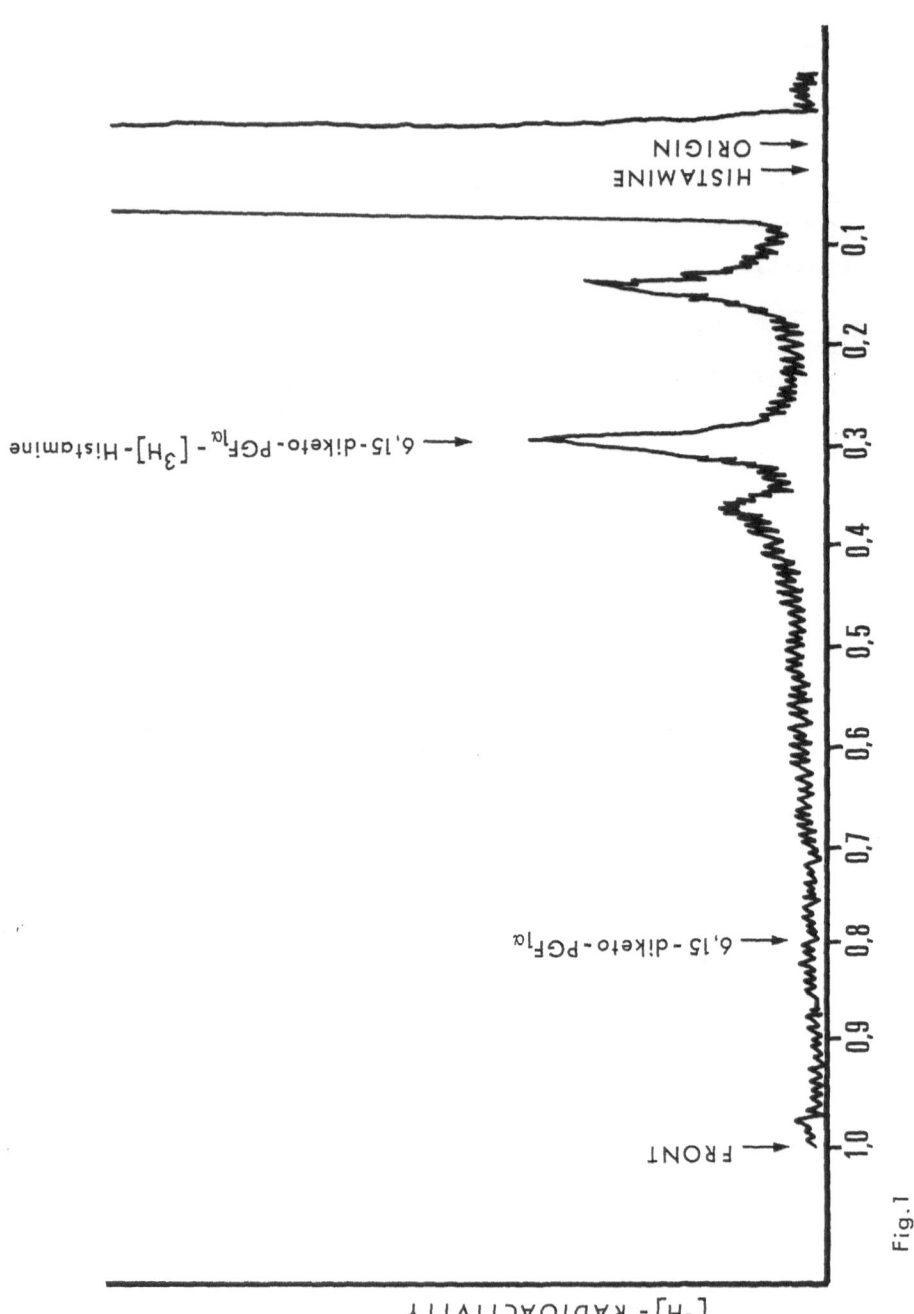

Fig. 1

37

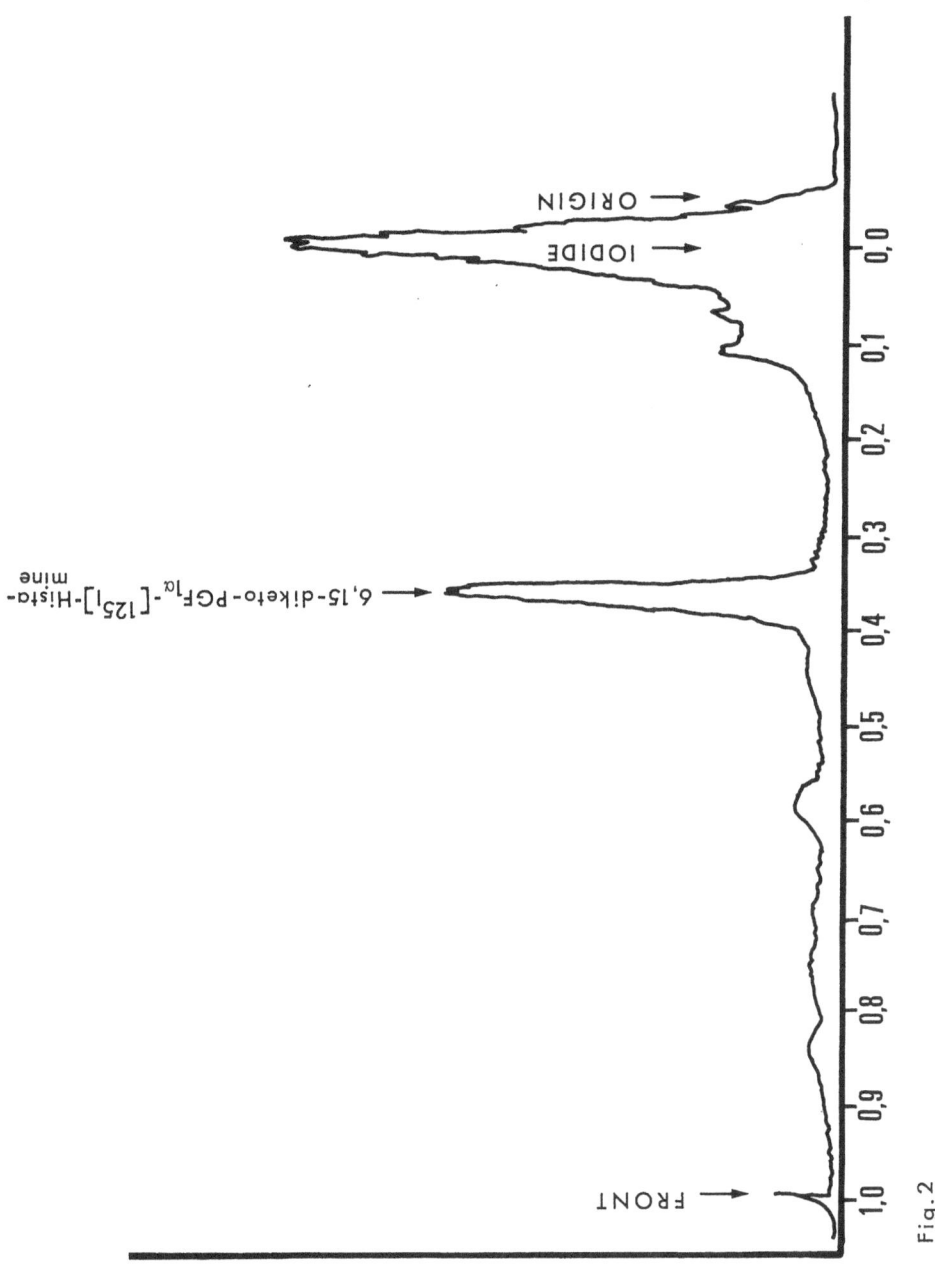

Fig. 2

38

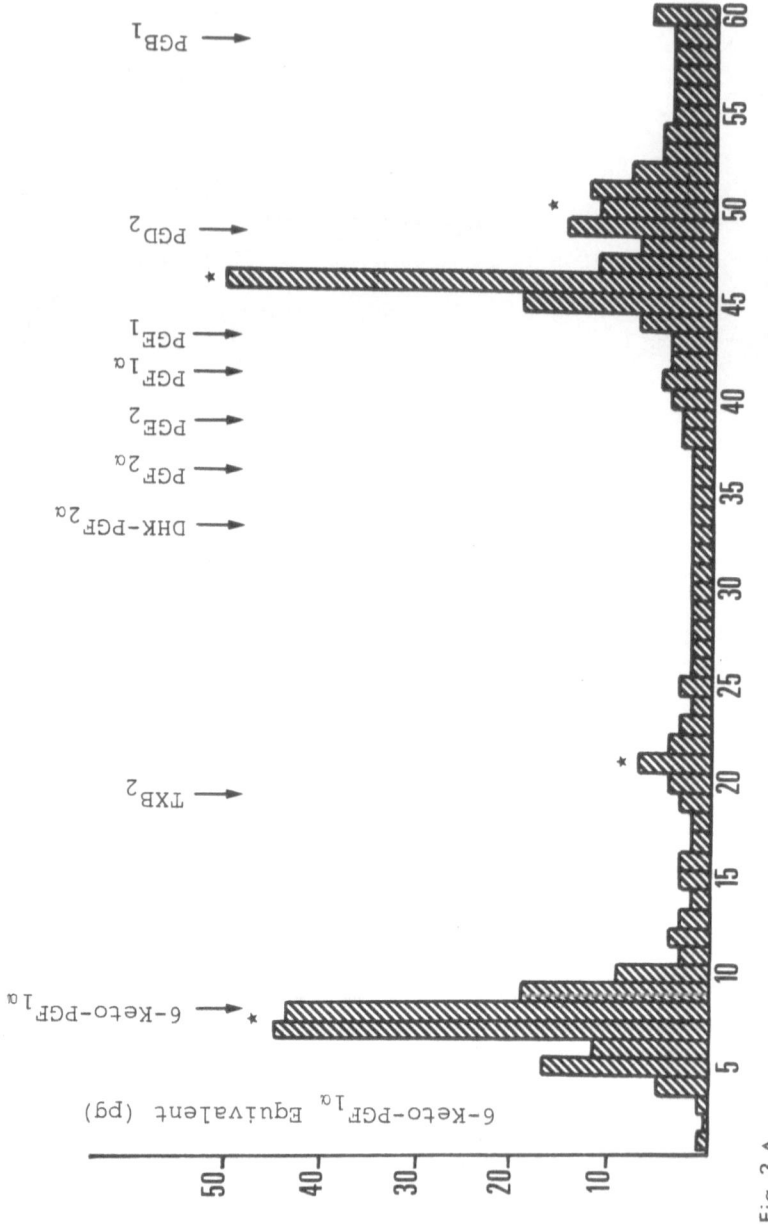

Fig. 3 A

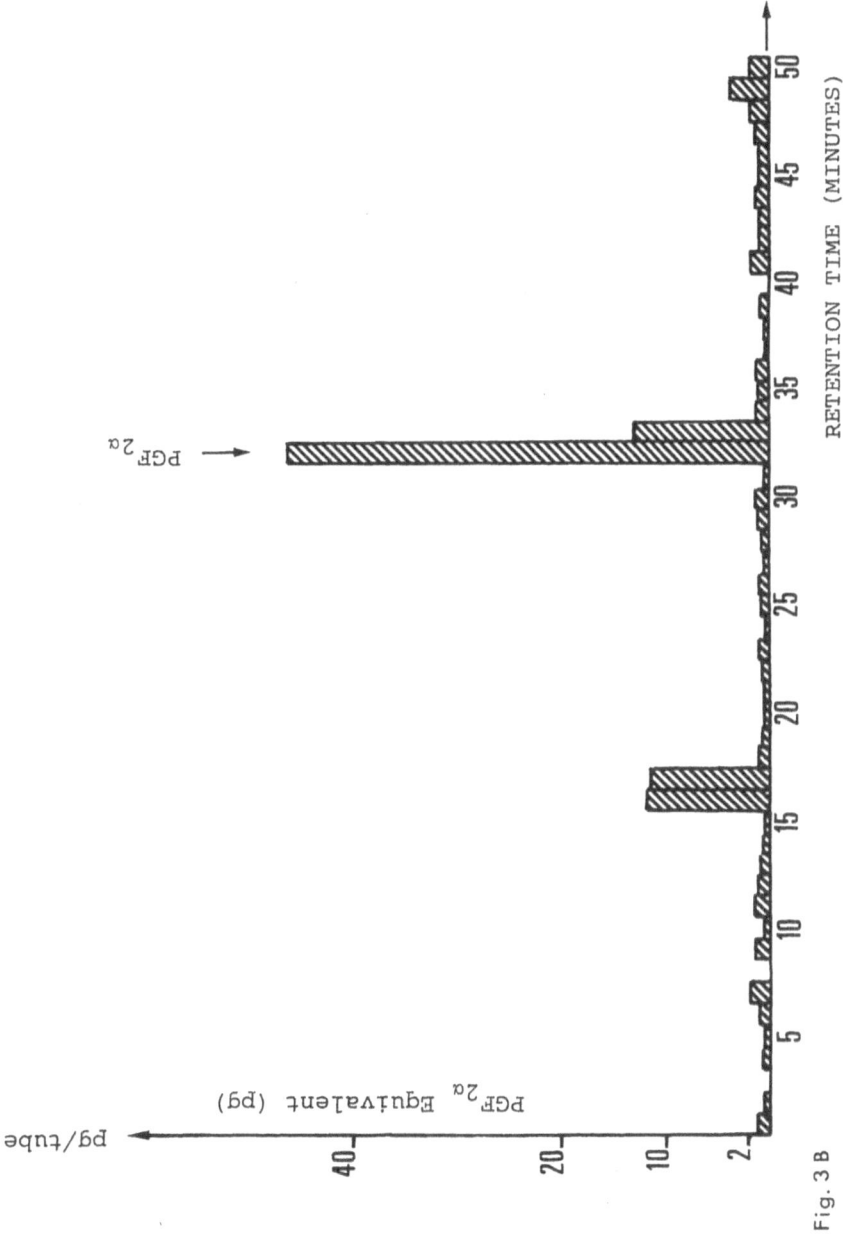

Fig. 3 B

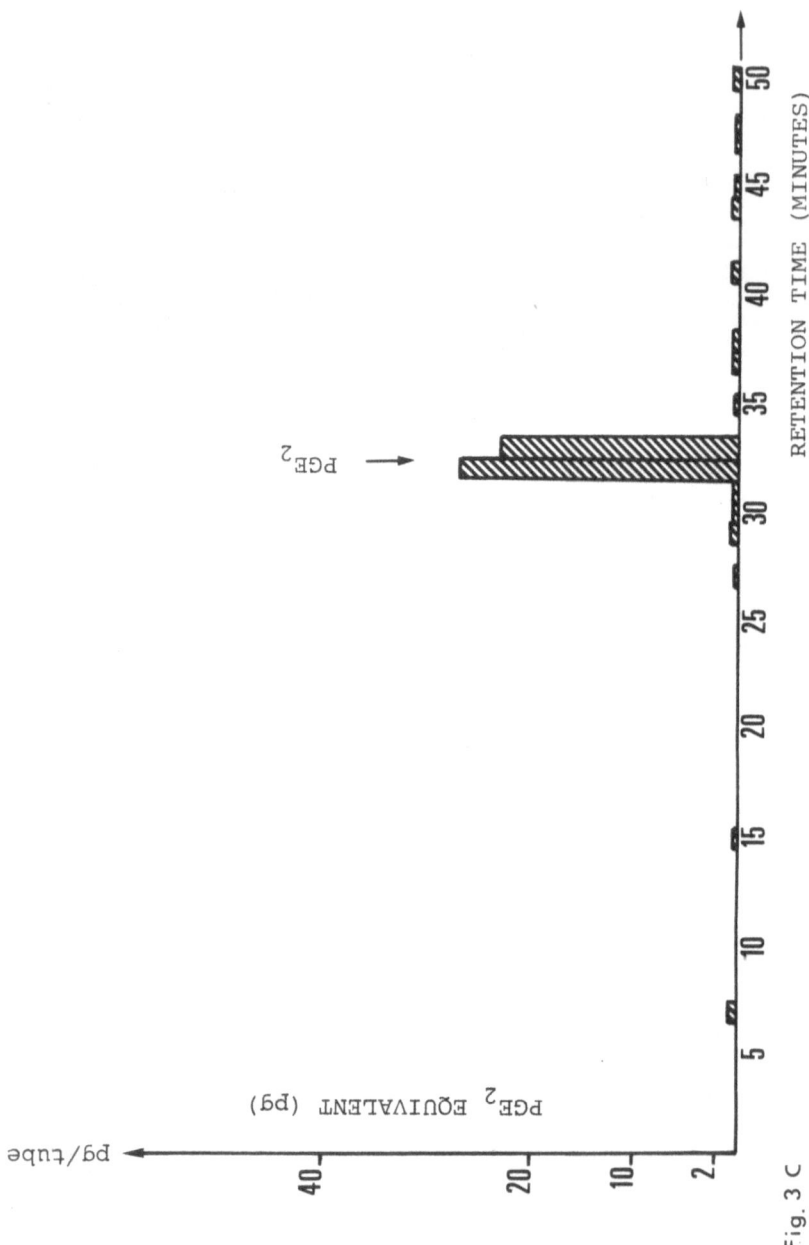

Fig. 3 C

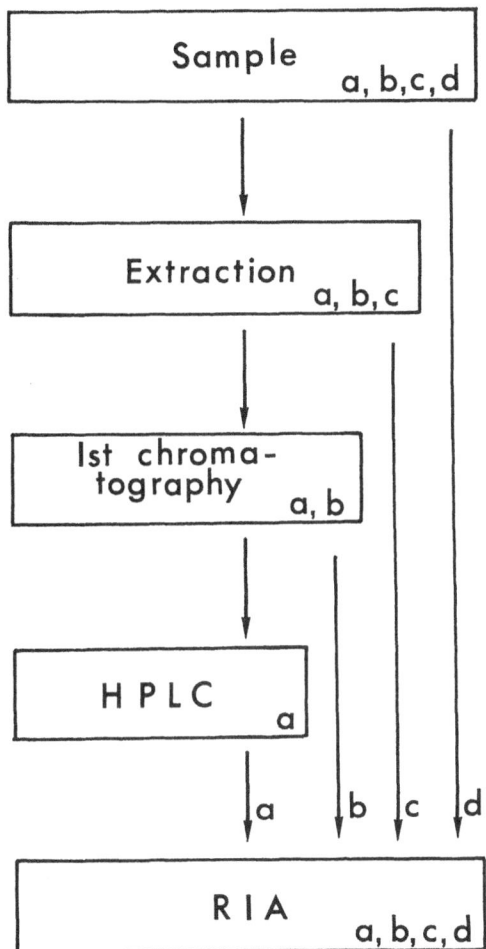

BIOLOGICAL MATERIAL

Critical step for any
quantitative analysis
of prostanoic derivatives
(as bio-assay, GC-MS, RIA ...)

Sample   a, b, c, d

Extraction   a, b, c

1st chroma-
tography   a, b

H P L C   a

a   b   c   d

R I A   a, b, c, d

HPLC : High Performance Liquid Chromatography
RIA : Radioimmunoassay

Fig. 4

42

DISCUSSION

J. Salmon Professor Dray's remarks about the use of iodinated derivatives instead of tritiated tracers for radioimmunoassays are becoming more
relevant. The use of these ^{125}I-derivatives are recommended not
only because they offer more sensitivity and are more economic but
also because various authorities are now introducing legislation
which will restrict the use of long lasting radioactive isotopes such
as tritium. Already, Frank Fitzpatrick has informed me that several
dumps for disposal of tritium have been closed down in the States.
Probably most of us have been lazy and if we can purchase tritiated
PGS from commercial sources we prefer to do that rather than performing a iodination every month or two. Another factor may be
that we consider that the iodination itself is a difficult procedure.
In our laboratory, we have used the Chlorium T method described
by Professor Dray with reasonable success but now prefer to use a
procedure using Iodogen$^{(R)}$(Pierce Chemical Company). I should
like to illustrate this procedure with two slides :

Iodination of PG-tyrosine methyl ester using Iodogen

Iodogen $\equiv$ (1,3,4,6-tetrachloro-3a,6a-diphenylglycoluril)

(1) 2µg Iodogen in dichloromethane (20µl) added to
plastic Ependorf tube.
(2) Dichloromethane carefully evaporated.
(3) PG-TME in 25µl Tris buffer added to tube which
gently shaken for 10min at room temperature.
(4) Add 200µCi Na^{125}I, reaction continued for
10min.
(5) Iodinated PG-TME purified by TLC.

Advantages of Procedure

(i) Very simple and practical.
(ii) Mild reaction - little danger of oxidising the
PG-TME conjugate.
(iii) Addition of reducing agent is unnecessary.
(iv) Single iodinations predominate.

TLC Purification of ^{125}I-Tyrosine Methyl Ester derivatives of:-

a) 6-keto-PGF$_{1\alpha}$ b) 6,15-diketo-PGF$_{1\alpha}$

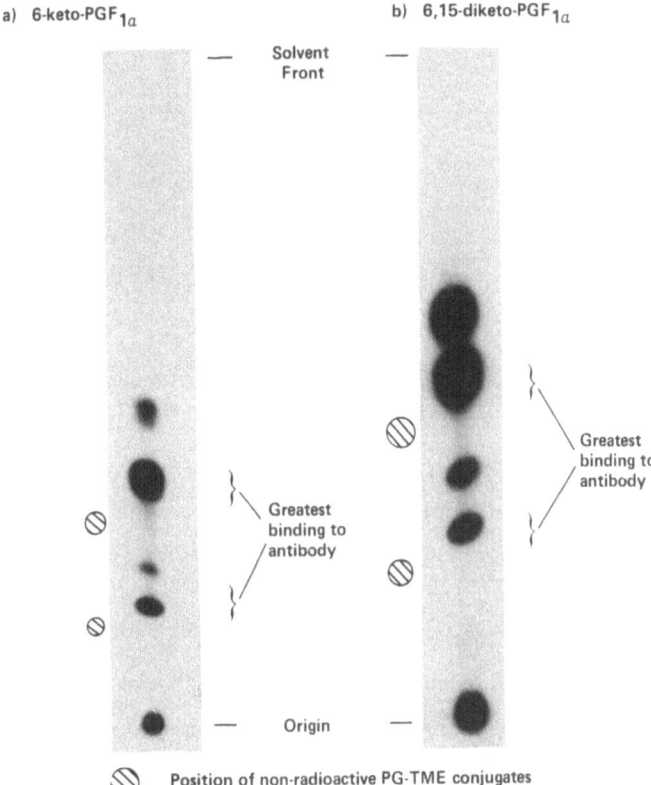

— Solvent Front —

Greatest binding to antibody

Greatest binding to antibody

Greatest binding to antibody

— Origin —

⬛ Position of non-radioactive PG-TME conjugates

As you can see the procedure is simple and the timings are not critical. There is no need to add reducing agent, the procedure is very mild (which makes the procedure eminently suitable for labelling proteins and polypeptides besides these prostaglandin conjugates) and monoiodinations predominate.

The purification by TLC illustrated on the second slide is similar to that already described by Professor Dray. We consider that the two spots of radioactivity which are well bound by antibody are due to variations in the structure of the 6-keto-PGF$_{1\alpha}$ or 6,15-diketo-PGF$_{1\alpha}$ (i.e. tautomers) rather than different isomers of the conjugate.

J. Salmon   I agree that TLC purification is not as efficient as silicic acid column chromatography (in our hands the recovery by TLC is about 50% of that obtained after silicic acid chromatography) but the TLC extract does contain specifically one prostaglandin or thromboxane and when we use Whatman LKD plates we do not have a "blank" problem.

3 DEVELOPMENT AND USE OF A RADIOIMMUNOASSAY FOR MEASURING 6-OXO-PROSTAGLANDIN $F_{1\alpha}$

N.L. Poyser

A) Introduction

Prostaglandins (PG) produced by the uterus have several roles in reproduction, for example, luteolysis, menstruation, implantation and parturition. Up to 1976, all the experimental evidence indicated that the major prostaglandin produced by the uterus was $PGF_{2\alpha}$ (1). However, studies on the pseudopregnant rat uterus around that time revealed that $6\text{-oxo-PGF}_{1\alpha}$, now known to be the more stable metabolite of prostacyclin ($PGI_{1\alpha}$), was the major prostaglandin synthesised by the broken cell preparation (2). For our studies on the uterus, therefore, it became essential to develop an assay for measuring $6\text{-oxo-PGF}_{1\alpha}$ accurately and precisely. This paper described the development of a radioimmunoassay (RIA) for measuring $6\text{-oxo-PGF}_{1\alpha}$. Parts of this work have been reported previously (3,4).

B) Raising of Antibodies
1) Preparation of $6\text{-oxo-PGF}_{1\alpha}$ Conjugate

$6\text{-oxo-PGF}_{1\alpha}$ (5 mg) was conjugated to 16.2 mg thyrogobulin using 1-ethyl-3-(3-dimethylaminopropyl) carbodiimide in aqueous solution at pH 5.5. The reaction took place at room temperature and lasted 5 hr. At the end of the reaction period, the solution was dialysed at 4 °C against, in succession, 200 ml 0.5 N sodium carbonate for 2 hr. (3 times), 200 ml 0.03 M phosphate buffer for 4 hr. (twice), and running water overnight. The retentate was suspended in 0.03 M sodium carbonate and centrifuged. The supernatant liquid was poured off and freeze-dried, to produce the dry conjugate. By incorporating 3 μCi $^3\text{H-PGF}_{2\alpha}$ in the reaction mixture, it was calculated that about 60 moles of PG became attached to 1 mole of thyroglobulin.

2) Immunization of Rabbits

Four rabbits (2 male and 2 female) were used. 4 mg 6-oxo-PGF$_{1\alpha}$ conjugate were dissolved in 4 ml sterile, normal saline and an emulsion formed with 4 ml Freund's complete adjuvant. 2 ml of this emulsion were injected intradermally at several sites on the shaved back of each rabbit. Booster injections were given subcutaneously every 6 to 12 weeks. 50 ml blood were collected 8 days after each boosting. The blood was allowed to clot and stored at 4 °C overnight. The serum obtained was centrifuged at 1000 g for 15 min, decomplemented by heating at 56 °C for 30 min, and, following the addition of sodium azide (0.1 mg/ml) as preservative, was dispensed into 2 aliquot samples and stored at -20 °C.

3) Preparation of ^{3}H-6-oxo-PGF$_{1\alpha}$

At the time of setting up this assay, ^{3}H-6-oxo-PGF$_{1\alpha}$ was not commercially available. It was decided, therefore, to synthesise ^{3}H-6-oxo-PGF$_{1\alpha}$ from ^{3}H-arachidonic acid, necessitating the development of a 6-oxo-PGF$_{1\alpha}$ synthesising system. An acetone-dried, microsomal preparation obtained from the sheep uterus proved highly satisfactory for this purpose. 25 mCi octa-tritiated arachidonic acid (sp. act. 120 Ci/mmol, Amersham, England) was reacted with 200 mg sheep uterus microsomes in 5 ml Krebs' solution (containing 1 mg/ml tryptophan and 10 μg/ml haemoglobin) aerated with 5% carbon dioxide in oxygen, at 37° C for 60 min. The acidity of the solution was then lowered to pH 4.5, and the prostaglandins extracted with ethyl acetate. The extract was evaporated to dryness, redissolved in 67% ethanol, and washed twice with petroleum ether (b.p. 60 to 80 °C) to remove unreacted ^{3}H-arachidonic acid. The ethanolic fraction was taken to dryness, and the residue was further purified by straight-phase, liquid-gel partition, column chromatography on Lipidex 1000. The column was eluted with hexane, 1,2 dichloroethane, ethanol, and acetic acid in the ratio of 100:100:15:0.2. Fractions of 3 ml were collected and the major peak of radioactivity occurred in fractions 16,17 and 18. These fractions were bulked, evaporated to dryness and the residue further purified by reversed-phase, high performance liquid chromatography. The column was packed with Partisil ODS, and was eluted with acetonitrile, water and acetic acid in the ratio of 40:60:0.1. The major radioactive substance isolated co-chromatographed with authentic 6-oxo-PGF$_{1\alpha}$ in two solvent systems, namely F VI (5) and 1a (6). The specific activity of the ^{3}H-6-oxo-PGF$_{1\alpha}$ prepared was 90 to 105 Ci/mmol depending on whether 1 or 2 tritium atoms had been lost during the reaction procedure.

4) Testing of Antisera

All rabbits produced antibodies to 6-oxo-PGF$_{1\alpha}$. The best anti-serum was obtained from rabbit No. 1, bleed 6, and this bound 60% of ^{3}H-6-oxo-PGF$_{1\alpha}$ (20 pg) at a dilution of 1:13000. Initially, 0.05 M phosphate buffer at pH 7.5 (containing 1 g/2 gelatin and 0.1 g/2 sodium azide) was used as diluent for the radioimmunoassay. Subsequently, it was found that more consistent results were obtained if tris-hydrochloride buffer at pH 6.8 (containing 1 g/L gelatin and 0.1 g/L sodium azide) was used. The cross reactivities of the antiserum from rabbit No. 1, bleed 6, in both diluents against other prostaglandins are shown in table 1. The cross-reactivities tended to be lower in the tris-hydrochloride diluent than in the phosphate diluent. PGE$_2$, PGE$_1$ and PGF$_{2\alpha}$ were the only sub-stances found to cross-react to any significance, but these were considered low enough to enable use of the antiserum for specifically measuring 6-oxo-PGF$_{1\alpha}$. The method of radioimmunoassay used was as described previously for other antisera raised in this laboratory (7), using the double-antibody method of separation.

C) Assay Procedure

1) Efficiency of Extraction

Lowering the acidity of aqueous solutions to between pH 4.0 and 4.5 with mineral or organic acid, followed by partitioning the aqueous solution 3 times with 2 volumes of ethyl acetate is a well-established method for efficiently extracting PGE_2 and $PGF_{2\alpha}$ (> 90% recovery). This extraction procedure, however, was found to be less efficient at extracting 6-oxo-$PGF_{1\alpha}$ from aqueous medium. Between pH 1.5 and 4.5, only 65% to 75% of added ^3H-6-oxo-$PGF_{1\alpha}$ (in the presence of 1 µg of 6-oxo-$PGF_{1\alpha}$) was extracted from Krebs' solution by ethyl acetate (table 2). The reasons for this lower recovery are not known. As this method of extraction has been used routinely for extracting 6-oxo-$PGF_{1\alpha}$ along with other prostaglandins from aqueous solutions, it must be borne in mind, therefore, that recovery of 6-oxo-$PGF_{1\alpha}$ is about 20% lower than the recovery of other prostaglandins when assessing the results.

2) Assessment of the accuracy and precision

The accuracy of the assay was assessed by adding known amounts of 6-oxo-$PGF_{1\alpha}$ (200,500 and 1000 ng) to 20 ml Krebs' solution, lowering the acidity of the solution to pH 3.5 or pH 4 with NHCl, extracting the prostaglandins with ethyl acetate, and then measuring the amounts recovered by radioimmunoassay. The values obtained were corrected for a mean recovery of 65%, and are shown in table 3. Close agreement was obtained between the "added" amount and the corrected "recovered" amount, showing that the assay can measure 6-oxo-$PGF_{1\alpha}$ accurately. In addition, a standard solution of 640 ng/ml 6-oxo-$PGF_{1\alpha}$ assayed in 8 consecutive assays gave a mean assay ($\pm$ s.e.m.) of 638 $\pm$ 31 ng/ml, with an interassay coefficient of variation of 13.5%. The intra-assay coefficient of variation was 12.4%, though both these coefficients of variation

48

were measured using phosphate diluent. Lower values nearer 10% are obtained if tris-hydrochloride diluent is used. The lower limit of detection for the assay ranges from 25 to 40 pg. The accuracy and precision of the assay were considered satisfactory for the assay of $6\text{-oxo-PGF}_{1\alpha}$.

D)   Use of the assay

$6\text{-oxo-PGF}_{1\alpha}$ production by incubations of homogenised rat uterus and ovaries has been measured on each day of the oestrous cycle (4). Production by the uterus was highest on day 1 and lowest on day 3 of the 4-day cycle. There was no daily variation in production by the ovary. For both tissues, $6\text{-oxo PGF}_{1\alpha}$ was the major prostaglandin synthesised.

$6\text{-oxo-PGF}_{1\alpha}$ was also found to be the major prostaglandin produced by homogenates of pseudopregnant and pregnant rat uterus, and the results obtained by both RIA and gas chromatography - mass spectrometry showed close agreement (C A Phillips and N L Poyser, unpublished results). Homogenates of the sheep myometrium also synthesised $6\text{-oxo-PGF}_{1\alpha}$ as the major production, whereas, in the endometrium, $PGF_{2\alpha}$ production exceeded $6\text{-oxo-PGF}_{1\alpha}$ production (S.N. Alwachi, K.P. Bland and N.L Poyser, unpublished results).

It is clear that the raising of antibodies to $6\text{-oxo-PGF}_{1\alpha}$ in rabbits and the use of this antisera for measuring $6\text{-oxo-PGF}_{1\alpha}$ by the uterus has been successful. The radioimmunoassay developed should also prove useful in measuring $6\text{-oxo-PGF}_{1\alpha}$ production by other tissues.

Acknowledgements

These studies were supported by the M.R.C. $6\text{-oxo-PGF}_{1\alpha}$ was kindly supplied by I.C.I. Pharmaceuticals Division, Cheshire, and Upjohn Company, Kalamazoo, U.S.A. The co-operation of Dr. K.K. Dighe, Dr. N.H. Wilson and Dr. R.L. Jones is acknowledged, and the technical assistance of Mr. C.G. Marr, Miss Agnes Pelanis, Miss Lynne Gilchrist, Miss Sylvia North and Miss Fiona Howson is appreciated.

References

1. Horton EW, Poyser NL: Uterine luteolytic hormone: A physiological role for prostaglandin $F_{2\alpha}$. Phys Rev (56):595-651, 1976.

2. Fenwick L, Jones RL, Naylor B, Poyser NL, Wilson NH: Production of prostaglandins by the pseudopregnant rat uterus, in vitro, and the effect of tamoxifen, with the identification of 6-keto-prostaglandin $F_{1\alpha}$ as a major product. Br J Pharmac (59):191-199, 1977.

3. Dighe KK, Jones RL, Poyser, NL: Development of a radioimmuno-assay for measuring 6-oxo-prostaglandin $F_{1\alpha}$. Br J Pharmac (63):406P, 1978.

4. Poyser NL, Scott, FM: Prostaglandin production by the rat uterus and ovary during the oestrous cycle, in vitro. J Reprod Fert, submitted for publication.

5. Anderson NH: Preparative thin-layer and column chromatography of prostaglandins. J Lip Res (10):316-319, 1969.

6. Cottee F, Flower RJ, Moncada S, Salmon JA, Vane JR: Synthesis of 6-keto-PGF$_{1\alpha}$ by ram seminal vesicle microsomes. Prostaglandins (14):413-423, 1977.

7. Dighe KK, Emslie HA, Henderson LK, Rutherford F, Simon L: The development of antisera to prostaglandins β_2 and $F_{2\alpha}$ and their analysis using solid-phase and double antibody radio-immunoassay methods. Br J Pharmac (55):503-514, 1975.

Table 1.   Results of cross-reactivity studies.

Compound	Percentage cross-reactivity of antiserum raised against 6-oxo-PGF-1α in:	
	Tris-hydrochloride Diluent	Phosphate Diluent
PGF-2α	4.0	5.8
PGE-2	4.2	6.8
PGD-2	< 0.01	0.073
PGA-2	0.065	0.036
PGB-2	0.03	0.031
6-oxo-PGF-1α	100	100
TXB-2	< 0.01	0.003
PGF-1α	0.43	0.12
PGE-1	1.1	2.0
15-oxo-PGF-2α	0.04	-
15-oxo-PGE-2	0.08	-
13,14-dihydro-15-oxo-PGF-2α	0.065	0.105
13,14-dihydro-15-oxo-PGE-2	0.09	0.018

Table 2.   An assessment of the accuracy of the radioimmunoassay

for measuring 6-oxo-PGF$_{1\alpha}$.   (n = 3 per group).

Amount added (ng).	Mean $\pm$ s.e.m. amount recovered (ng, corrected for a 65% recovery) following extraction at:-	
	pH 3.5	pH 4.0
200	191 $\pm$ 23	229 $\pm$ 13
500	521 $\pm$ 26	496 $\pm$ 28
1000	973 $\pm$ 35	976 $\pm$ 38

Table 3.   Percentage recovery of ^{3}H-6-oxo-PGF$_{1\alpha}$ (0.5 μCi) from 10 ml Krebs' solution (containing 1 μg of 6-oxo-PGF$_{1\alpha}$) by ethyl acetate at acid pH.

pH of Krebs' solution	% recovery ^{3}H-6-oxo-PGF$_{1\alpha}$ (mean $\pm$ s.e.m.; n = 3)
1.5	67.4 $\pm$ 1.3
2.0	65.8 $\pm$ 2.9
2.5	66.6 $\pm$ 3.1
3.0	71.2 $\pm$ 1.6
3.5	65.7 $\pm$ 5.1
4.0	65.3 $\pm$ 1.2
4.5	63.4 $\pm$ 2.5
5.0	35.9 + 4.7

DISCUSSION

A. Herman	1. How long do your sheep uterus microsomes keep their ability to synthesize 6-keto-$PGF_{1\alpha}$?
	2. Do you systematically include a HPLC purification step for your RIA?
N. Poyser	1. I do not really know the stability of the enzyme since I have not studied this particular problem. I always prepared the enzyme and used it several days later.
	2. No.
J. Salmon	Away from methodology for one minute – do you have any evidence that there is an actual enzyme in the uterus which converts prostaglandin endoperoxides to $PGF\alpha$?
N. Poyser	I have not studied this particular problem but from the literature, it has not yet been demonstrated that such a specific enzyme exists in other tissues.
P. Lijnen	Did you check whether there is any difference in the plasma level of 6-oxo-$PGF_{1\alpha}$ assayed directly; after extraction with organic solvents and after chromato-graphic fractionation?
N. Poyser	I have not yet measured 6-oxo-$PGF_{1\alpha}$ in plasma samples.
E.Schell-Frederick	What is the cross reactivity with arachidonic acid in your assay?
N. Poyser	I do not know the exact figure, but it is very low, certainly less than 0.1 %.

F. Cattabeni — Before doing the recovery studies at the 6-keto-PGF$_{1\alpha}$ did you check the radioactive purity of the compound?

N. Poyser — I am certain the ^{3}H-6-oxo-PGF$_{1\alpha}$ was pure. It was purified extensively when I made it, and it worked well in the radioimmunoassay. If the ^{3}H-6-oxo-PGF$_{1\alpha}$ was deteriorating, this would show up in the assay by lower percentage binding.

H. Kindahl — Is it not possible that the low extraction recovery of 6-keto-PGF$_{1\alpha}$ is due to the formation of water soluble derivatives in the buffer, and if this is the case that large variation could be obtained when extracting different biological samples? Have you looked at the recoveries from e.g. water, different kinds of buffers, and different biological samples.

N. Poyser — 1. It is possible that a more polar product is formed. Obviously the % recovery of 6-oxo-PGF$_{1\alpha}$ in different biological systems needs to be studied. Hopefully, the recovery from the same biological system is fairly constant, but this can only be shown as we become more experienced with extracting and measuring 6-oxo-PGF$_{1\alpha}$

2. No.

M. Claeys — Could you give some details on the GC/MS method for measuring PGD$_2$? You find high levels of PGD$_2$ in the uterus. Is there any role for it?

N. Poyser — 1) PGD$_2$ was monitored by recording the ion at m/e 510 of the methyl ester butyloxime, trimethylsilyl ether derivative (Me-BO-TMS; when value of 2nd isomer = 26.1). The corresponding ethyl ester derivative of

PGD_2 (Et – BuO– TMS; when value of 2nd isomer =
26.4) was used as internal standard, and the ion at m/e
524 was recorded. Standard quantities of 5,10,20 and
40 ng PGD_2 (as Me–BuO–TMS) together with 40 ng
PGD_2 (as Et–BuO–TMS) were injected into the GC–MS
and the peak heights at 510 and 524 measured. A standard line was plotted of ratio of heights 510 ion to 524
ion against standard quantity of PGD_2.

2) I do not know of any roles really. It is weakly spasmo-
genic, but is a vasoconstrictor in the rat and sheep.

H. Seyberth
1) What is your feeling about indomethacin treatment in
pregnancy (e.g. to prevent premature contraction)?
2) What is your experience about stability of ^{3}H-6-keto-
$PGF_{1\alpha}$ in methanol?

N. Poyser
1) It has been recommended that indomethacin should not
be used since it can cross the placenta and cause con-
striction of the ductus arteriosus. This is particularly
important in the last trimester. Whether indomethacin
affects uterine and/or placental blood flow during
pregnancy in women is not known.

2) I find that ^{3}H-6-oxo-$PGF_{1\alpha}$ is quite stable when
stored in redistilled methanol at -20°C. For use, I eva-
porate off the methanol and dissolve the ^{3}H-6-oxo $PGF_{1\alpha}$
in the appropriate aqueous medium.

4 A COMPARISON BETWEEN BIOLOGIC, RADIOIMMUNOLOGIC AND MASS SPECTROMETRIC ANALYSIS OF PROSTAGLANDINS

F. Cattabeni, S. Nicosia, G.C. Folco, D. Longiave and R. Paoletti

1. INTRODUCTION

Many analytical problems arise when sensitivity has to be combined with specificity, as in the determination of arachidonic acid metabolites. In fact, the analytical method required for the analysis of these compounds must be sensitive, due to the very low levels of Prostaglandins (PGs) in body fluids and tissues. On the other hand, the method must be specific in order to avoid interferences in the measurement of a single PG; such interferences can arise from other PGs or from chemically related compounds (other insaturated fatty acids) present in the same tissues. Several different methods have been set up and are utilized for PGs determinations: Bioassay, Radioimmunoassay (RIA) and Mass Fragmentography (MF) are among those commonly used.

Each of these methods has advantages and disadvantages which will be discussed here and which must be taken into consideration before a choice is made on which method to use.

Moreover, we will also report on the data obtained for the measurement of $PGF_{2\alpha}$ and PGE_2 subjecting the same samples to Bioassay, RIA and MF. Samples analyzed were rat brain cortex and human urine.

2. BIOASSAY, RIA AND MASS FRAGMENTOGRAPHY: ADVANTAGES AND DISADVANTAGES IN PGs MEASUREMENT.

Table 1 lists the advantages and the disadvantages of these methods in PGs measurement. We wish to point out that this discussion applies only to the specific problem of PG level evaluation and it cannot be applied as such

Table 1. Advantages and disadvantages of RIA, Mass Fragmentography and Bioassay for the measurement of arachidonic acid metabolites.

	ADVANTAGES	DISADVANTAGES
RIA	1. Low cost 2. High number of samples 3. Simple equipment 4. High sensitivity	1. Danger connected to the use of Radioisotopes 2. Different assay for each compound present in the same sample 3. Possible interference by unknown compounds
MASS FRAGMENT.	1. High specificity 2. Several compounds analyzed simoultaneously 3. High versatility 4. Response linear over a wide range (1— 1000)	1. High costs, sophisticated equipment 2. Low number of samples can be analyzed 3. Sensitivity lower than RIA
BIOASSAY	1. Low cost 2. New compounds can be detected 3. Several compounds can be analyzed in cascade 4. Immediate response (possibility of detecting unstable compounds)	1. Sensitivity lower than RIA 2. Quantitation approximate 3. Low specificity

to the measurement of other endogenous compounds and is not valid in general terms.

2.1. *RIA:*

This method is today generally used for routine measurement of PGs and related compounds (1,2). In fact, once the method has been set up, the cost is relatively lower than MF, the equipment needed to perform the analysis is rather simple to use and a large number of samples can be analyzed with an excellent sensitivity (limit of detection 10^{-12} g). RIA is the ideal method for routine analysis of PGs. The major disadvantage of this technique is the use of radioactive isotopes, although immunoassays with non radioactive tracers (EIA, ELISA) are under development for a number of compounds. Moreover, if more than one compound must be measured in the same sample, separate assays have to be performed.

2.2. *Mass fragmentography:*

This method is considered to be one of the most specific ones, since the measurement is based upon the chemical structure of the compound to be determined. This does not exclude the possibility of interfering compounds, especially when dealing with biological samples, as it will be shown later. However the major advantage of MF is its high versatility. Not only mass spectrometry is very useful in identifying new arachidonic acid metabolites, but it can be adapted rather easily to the quantitative measurement of these new compounds. Moreover, MF allows for the simoultaneous measurement of more than one PG in the same sample and during the same analysis (3). Finally, it must be pointed out that with MF there is another definite advantage: the possibility to use an internal standard. If the internal standard is added to the sample at the beginning of the purification procedure, there is no need for recovery correction.

Perhaps the major disadvantage of MF is due to the high cost of the equipment and - more important and critical - the need of skilled personnel to perform the instrumental analysis.

Compared to RIA, relatively fewer samples can be analyzed and the sensitivity is about one order of magnitude lower (limit of detection 10^{-11} g).

2.3. *Bioassay:*

This method has been extensively utilized for PGs measurements and in fact the whole PGs field has been opened up with the help of Bioassay (4). The major advantage of it is that compounds with a very short half life can be measured if the preparation has been done properly. This is not possible with RIA and MF, since both these methods entail previous purification of the sample.

Bioassay has a relatively low cost and more than one compound can be measured in the same sample if organs with different sensitivities to the different compounds are mounted on cascade. On the other hand the sensitivity, at least for PGE_2 and $PGF_{2\alpha}$ is a little lower than RIA, as it will be described later.

The disadvantages of the bioassay are due to its specificity, which is definitely lower than that of MF and perhaps, also than that of RIA. However, it must be kept in mind that RIA can be considered a bioassay, since it is based on a biological response that is the immune reaction. Finally, the quantitation with bioassay is less accurate than with the other two methods. The above considerations stem from the results obtained by measuring $PGF_{2\alpha}$ and PGE_2 with the three different methods in the same samples of rat brain cortex and human urine.

3. COMPARATIVE MEASUREMENTS OF $PGF_{2\alpha}$.

3.1. *Rat brain cortex.*

The scheme of the sample workup is described in Table 2.

As first instance, it must be emphasized that a reliable measurement of arachidonic acid metabolites in

Table 2. Sample workup for comparative PG measurement in rat brain cortex.

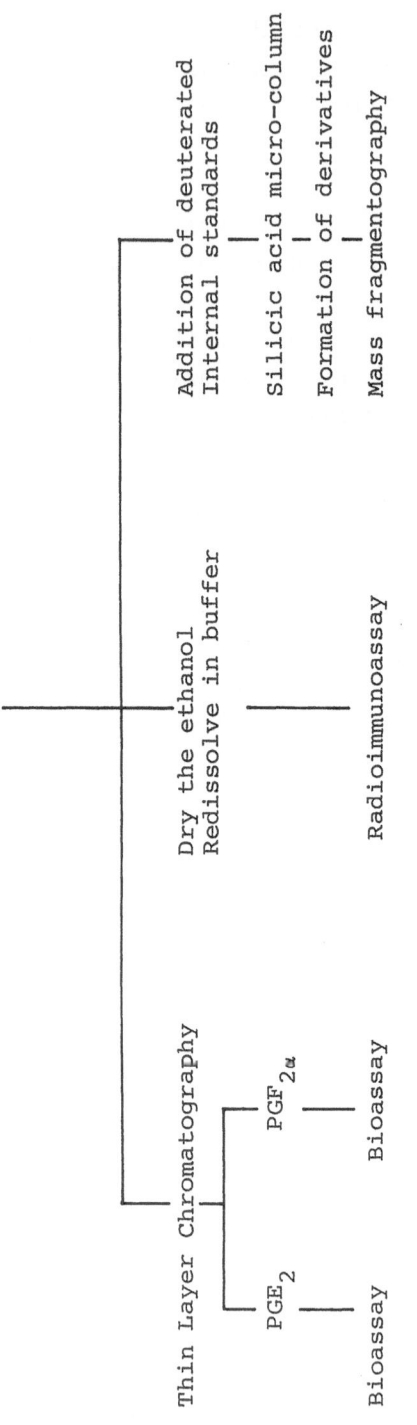

- Sacrifice the animals with high energy microwave irradiation
- Remove brain cortex
- Homogenize in absolute ethanol
- Centrifuge at 0°C for 30 min at 3000 x g

Dry the ethanol
Redissolve in buffer

Thin Layer Chromatography

PGE$_2$ PGF$_{2\alpha}$

Bioassay   Bioassay

Radioimmunoassay

Addition of deuterated Internal standards

Silicic acid micro-column

Formation of derivatives

Mass fragmentography

brain is obtained only if the animals are killed by high energy microwave irradiation. Only this procedure prevents post-mortem changes due to its ability to instantaneously inactivity brain enzymes. Guillottine sacrifice produces brain ischemia and artifactual increase of arachidonic acid metabolites concentrations (5).

Sample manipulation was identical for the three methods only up to the separation of precipitated proteins from the supernatant in absolute ethanol. Quite different procedures were than applied to different aliquots of this supernatant. For RIA, no further purification steps were required. However, mass fragmentographic analysis showed that interfering compounds are present if the sample is not previously purified on a silicic acid column. Losses due to this step are corrected by the previous addition of the deuterated internal standard. On the other hand, bioassay requires that the different PGs are separated on thin layer chromatography in order to confer specificity to the measurement.

Individual techniques have been previously described in detail (6). The results obtained measuring $PGF_{2\alpha}$ with the three methods in rat brain cortex are shown in Fig. 1. It can be noted that levels found are practically identical not only in control animals, but also in animals receiving 100 mg/kg of a compound known to stimulate PG synthesis. It is important that methods are validated also in animals which have undergone pharmacological treatment: in fact the possibility that under such treatment cross reacting metabolites are formed, cannot be excluded "a priori". This holds true not only for RIA or Bioassay, but also for mass fragmentography. Levels of $PGF_{2\alpha}$ in animals receiving 50 mg/kg of pentamethylenetetrazole are also shown in Fig. 1. Also in this case the agreement between RIA and mass fragmentography is excellent. Bioassay was not performed on these samples.

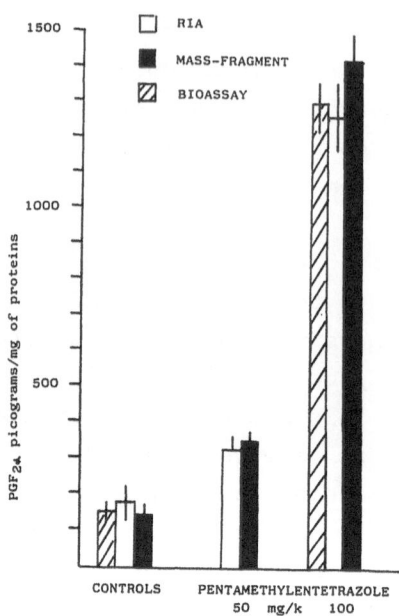

Fig. 1. *PGF$_{2\alpha}$ levels in brain cortex of control and penta-methylentetrazole treated rats measured by RIA, Mass fragmentography and Bioassay.*

3.2. *Human urine:*

Samples of 25 ml of human urine were processed as described in Table 3. Due to the higher number of interfering compounds present in these samples, even RIA required a purification step previous to the assay. The results obtained with the three methods on 4 urine samples are reported in Table 4. As it can be seen, both RIA and Bioassay gave results higher of one order of magnitude compared with mass fragmentography. This indicates that the purification procedure did not remove an interfering compound which cross-reacted with both the antibody and the organ preparation used for the Bioassay. On the other hand, this unknown compound did not interfere with the mass fragmentographic assay. It must also be emphasized that this interference was not removed by thin layer chromatography, which was used before the bioassay to separate PGF$_{2\alpha}$ from PGE$_2$. Cross-reactivity of this interfering compound was not

Table 3. Sample workup for comparative PG measurement in human urine.

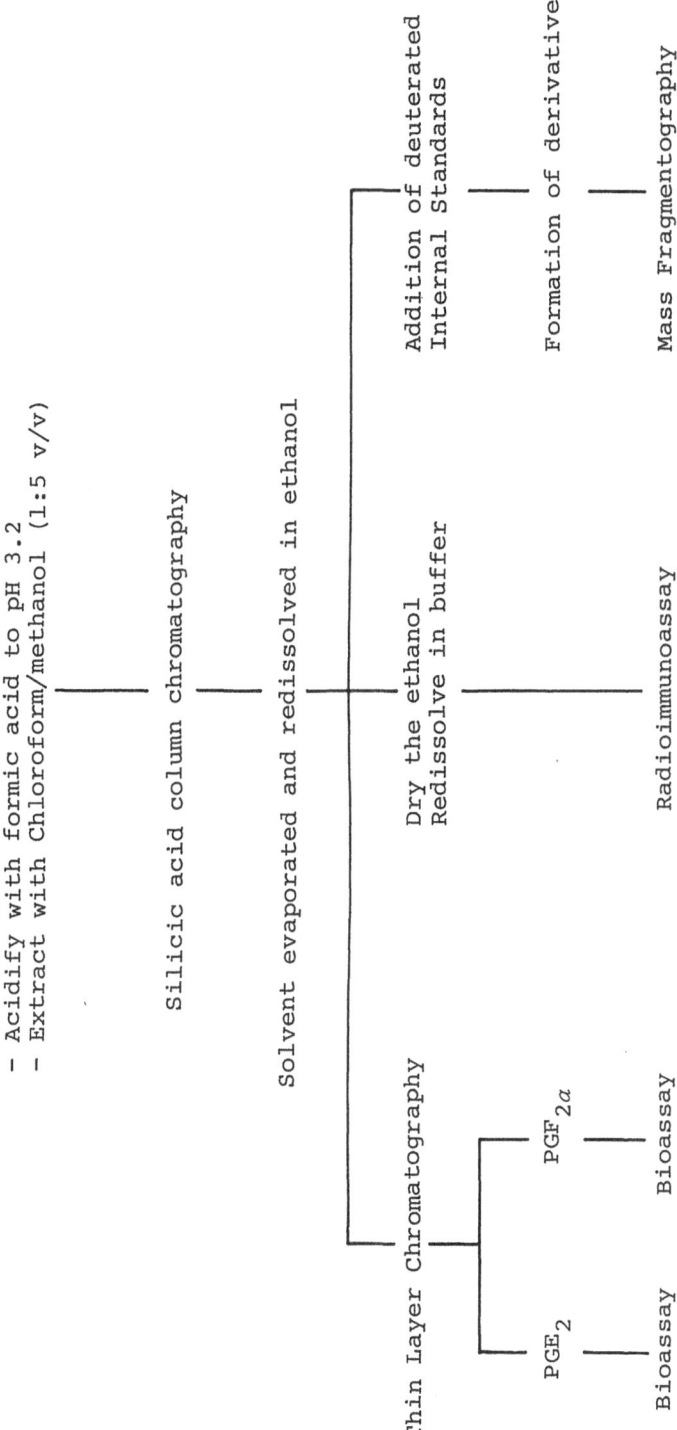

- Adjust 25 ml to pH 6.5 with NaOH
- Wash with benzene/1-Chlorobutane (1:1 v/v)
- Acidify with formic acid to pH 3.2
- Extract with Chloroform/methanol (1:5 v/v)

Silicic acid column chromatography

Solvent evaporated and redissolved in ethanol

Thin Layer Chromatography

PGE_2 $PGF_{2\alpha}$

Bioassay   Bioassay

Dry the ethanol
Redissolve in buffer

Radioimmunoassay

Addition of deuterated
Internal Standards

Formation of derivatives

Mass Fragmentography

Table 4. Comparative measurements of PGF$_{2\alpha}$ in human urine (ng/ml).

Sample No.	Mass Fragmentography	Bioassay	RIA
1	28.9	150[+]	179.5
2	12.2	150[+]	156.0
3	18.1	60	38.7
4	18.7	130	104.5

[+]*Signal out of scale. 150 pg of PGF$_{2\alpha}$ produced maximal response.*

observed if PGF$_{2\alpha}$ was measured by RIA utilizing a different antibody (2). The data reported in Table 5 clearly show that with this antibody the mass fragmentographic results are comparable with those obtained by RIA.

Table 5. Levels of PGF$_{2\alpha}$ (ng/ml) in human urine utilizing antibodies obtained in rabbits (I) and guinea pigs (II).

Sample No.	Antibody	
	I	II[+]
1	179.5	11.1
2	156.0	4.0
3	38.7	7.8
4	104.5	7.2

[+]*Antibody II was produced at the Institute of Pharmacology, Catholic University, Rome (see ref. 2).*

In order to better correlate RIA with mass fragmentography, urine samples of a patient with Bartter's syndrome before and after indomethacine treatment were analyzed. No bioassay was performed on these samples. Fig. 2 shows that an acceptable correlation exists between the levels measured with these two assays, provided that the second antibody against PGF$_{2\alpha}$ is used.

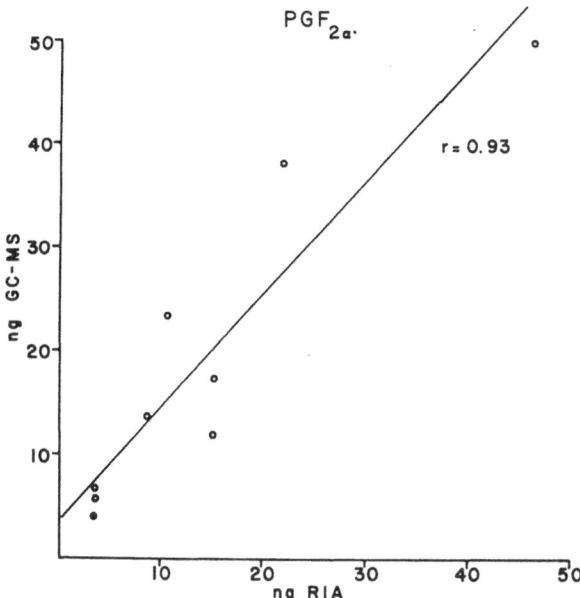

Fig. 2. Regression analysis of PGF$_{2\alpha}$ levels measured in human urine by Mass Fragmentography and RIA.

4. COMPARATIVE MEASUREMENTS OF PGE$_2$.

4.1. *Rat brain cortex.*

The same sample workup procedure described in Table 2 was used. The data reported in Tables 6 and 7 are raw data obtained in cortex samples of different weight. As it can be seen, MF, Bioassay and RIA gave results of the same order of magnitude. It must be noted, however, that the data for MF are in many cases about twice those obtained by the other methods. It is difficult to attribute a statistical significance to this discrepancy: it must be reminded, on the other hand, that only mass fragmentography is able to correct, for each sample, losses due to sample manipulation, since deuterated internal standards are added prior to purification of the sample.

Table 6. *Measurement of PGE$_2$ in rat brain cortex (total ng in sample): comparison of MF and Bioassay.*

Sample No.	MF	Bioassay
1	59.59	22.9
2	65.84	25.6
3	40.83	35.3
4	15.93	15.8

Table 7. *Measurement of PGE$_2$ in rat brain cortex (total ng in sample): comparison of MF and RIA[+].*

Sample No.	MF	RIA
5	4.00	1.80
6	33.74	12.60
7	8.98	6.75
8	26.50	19.60
9	5.19	2.94
10	4.64	6.70

[+]*RIA was performed at the Institute of Pharmacology, Catholic University, Rome (see ref. 2).*

4.2. *Human urine:*

In a first set of four samples of human urine the results obtained with the three methods are in excellent agreement (Table 8). Mass fragmentography proved to be a less sensitive method than Bioassay or RIA: in fact in two samples PGE$_2$ was below the detection limit, even if a larger aliquot of the ethanol extract was used for MF. On the other hand, these low levels were confirmed by RIA.

PGE$_2$ was measured also in the same human urine samples were PGF$_{2\alpha}$ was measured. In this case some samples showed high discrepancies between RIA and MF values (Table 9).

Table 8. *Comparative measurement of* PGE$_2$ *(ng/ml) in human urine.*

Sample No.	MF	RIA[+]	Bioassay
1	10.1	14.1	20.5
2	<1	0.5	2.2
3	<1	1.2	0.7
4	2.0	2.5	3.6

[+]*Assay performed at the Dept. of Pharmacology, Catholic University, Rome (see ref. 2).*

Table 9. *Comparative measurement of* PGE$_2$ *(ng/sample) in human urine.*

Sample	RIA[+]	Mass Fragmentography [++]	[+++]
1 Controls	24.8	72.14	61.3
2 "	1.89	11.10	0.26
3 Bartter's Syndrome	6.75	31.37	20.53
4 "	6.21	13.07	2.23
5 "	1.8	11.99	1.15
6 "	2.16	11.57	0.73
7 "	3.24	15.85	5.01
8 "	5.94	15.14	4.30
9 "	1.08	12.19	1.35
Blank	--	11.59	--
		10.84	
Blank	--	10.10	--

[+]*RIA was performed at the Institute of Pharmacology, Catholic University, Rome (see ref. 2)*

[++]*Without subtraction of the blank value.*

[+++]*With subtraction of the blank value.*

On the other hand, these samples contained a compound which interfered with PGE$_2$ analysis in our instrumental conditions. In fact, blank samples gave a signal corresponding to about 10 ng/sample of the Prostaglandin.

It has been suggested (1) that phtalic acid esters

could interfere in RIA of PGs, although cross-reactivity is present only at very high concentrations. On the other hand they pose more serious problems to the mass fragmentographic analysis. Therefore, any contact with plastic containers should be avoided for the mass fragmentographic analysis of PGs at the low nanogram level, since phtalates are commonly present in all types of plastic material.

5. CONCLUSIONS

PGs can be assayed successfully in different kind of samples either with Bioassay, RIA or Mass Fragmentography. With regard to sensitivity, RIA seems to be better than the other two assays on routine basis. The sensitivity reached by Mass Fragmentography is, on the other hand, dependent upon instrumental conditions. Sensitivities in the order of a few picograms can be obtained with instruments of the last generation and therefore no final conclusion on sensitivity must be drawn from the results reported in this paper.

What has to be borne in mind, is that RIA needs validation with a chemico-physical technique such as Mass Fragmentography. In fact, antibodies obtained in two different animals yield quite different results, when compared with those obtained by Mass Fragmentography, when analyzing $PGF_{2\alpha}$ in samples of different biological origin (Tables 6 and 7).

RIA can therefore be considered an excellent routine method for analyzing large numbers of samples: however, the specificity of the assay has to be controlled beforehand.

Mass Fragmentography is more versatile than RIA if new arachidonic acid metabolites are found for which an analytical technique has to be developed. No major problems are encountered to find the appropriate gas chromatographic and mass spectrometric conditions for compounds with a structure similar to that of PGs. The only real problem is represented by the availability of the appropriate internal standard. Since it is desirable that the internal standard is the deuterated analog of the compound to be measured, especially in view of the fact that extensive purification procedures are required due to the low levels of these compounds, the real problem is the synthesis of the deuterated analog. At the present time, the deuterated analogues of arachidonic acid metabolites are not commercially available: this fact hampers the use of mass fragmentography on a routine basis.

Bioassay should also be considered as a quantitative method in the PGs field. In fact this assay is particularly useful in determining chemically unstable compounds such as Thromboxane A_2 and PGI_2 (Prostacyclin). These compounds can be measured by Bioassay as soon as they are released, prior to their chemical transformation to more stable products, i.e. Thromboxane B_2 and 6-Keto-$PGF_{1\alpha}$. On the other hand, for PGs of the E and F series Bioassay seems to be of minor value due to the availability of the RIA. Moreover, Bioassay requires laborious and skillful preparation of the isolated organs.

We can therefore conclude that the three different techniques should be available to laboratories involved in arachidonic acid metabolites'studies: RIA for routine assays, Bioassay to measure unstable compounds and to reveale the presence of new active metabolites and Mass Fragmentography to validate the other assays and to develop in reasonable time quantitative assays for these new compounds.

6. ACKNOWLEDGEMENTS
This research has been supported by the CNR grant PF-TBM 79.01193.86

7. REFERENCES

1. Granström E: Sources of error in prostaglandin and Thromboxane radioimmunoassay. In: *Radioimmunoassay of Drugs
   and Hormones*, Albertini A, Da Prada M, Peskar BA (eds),
   Amsterdam-New York-Oxford, Elsevier/North Holland Biomedical Press, 1979, p 229-238.

2. Ciabattoni G, Pugliese F, Cinotti GA, Patrono C: Methodo-
   logic problems in the radioimmunoassay of prostaglandin
   E_2 and $F_{2\alpha}$ in human urine. In: *Radioimmunoassay of Drugs
   and Hormones*, Albertini A, Da Prada M, Peskar BA (eds),
   Amsterdam-New York-Oxford, Elsevier/North Holland Biomedical Press, 1979, p 265-280.

3. Nicosia S, Galli G: Vapor-phase methods for quantitative
   evaluation of prostaglandins and related compounds in
   biological samples. In: *Prostaglandins and Thromboxanes*,
   Berti F, Samuelsson B, Velo GP (eds), New York and
   London, 1977, p 53-63.

4. Moncada S, Ferreira SH, Vane JR: Bioassay of prostaglandins and biologically active substances derived from
   arachidonic acid. In: *Advance in Prostaglandin and
   Thromboxane Research*, vol. 5, Frölich JC (ed), New York,
   Raven Press, 1978, p 211-236.

5. Bosisio E, Galli C, Galli G, Nicosia S, Spagnuolo C, Tosi
   L: Correlation between release of free arachidonic acid
   and prostaglandin formation in brain cortex and cerebel-
   lum. *Prostaglandins* 11(5): 773-781, 1978.

6. Cattabeni F, Borghi C, Folco GC, Nicosia S, Spagnuolo C:
   RIA of $PGF_{2\alpha}$ and PGE_2 in biological samples of different
   origin: comparison with the mass fragmentographic technique. In: *Radioimmunoassay of Drugs and Hormones*,
   Albertini A, Da Prada M, Peskar BA (eds), Amsterdam-New
   York-Oxford, Elsevier/North Holland Biomedical Press,
   1979, p 281-289.

DISCUSSION

M. Korteweg   How did you separate the bound and free prostaglandins in your RIA of urine because the use of Norit for example, may give rise to your high levels with your (rabbit) anti PGF. With a second antibody (goat-anti rabbit) you may obtain lower levels.

F. Cattabeni   The bound and free was separated by centrifuging at 0°C for 30 min at 12,500 × g.

H. Seyberth   Do you think your clean up procedure is sufficient for GC-MS analysis? I don't think that just a simple open SiO_2-column will do it.

F. Cattabeni   I think that the clean up procedure is sufficient if we would get rid of plasticisers, in particular phtalates. In fact, as I showed, occasionally bad interference can occur. Usually, this happens if plastic containers are utilized for storing urine.

J. Salmon   Do you correct your bioassay (in combination with thin layer chromatography) results for procedural losses? Do you include tritiated PG's to assess recovery?

F. Cattabeni   Yes, all the results reported were recorded for losses due to TLC purification. These losses are around 30-40 %. This was established by a small tracer dose of ^{3}H-PG's.

M. Claeys   Another disadvantage you didn't mention is the availability of deuterated internal standards. The situation is not so bad for PGE_2 and F_2, for these we can obtain standards from Upjohn but is not so good for TXB_2 and 6-oxo $PGF_{1\alpha}$, for which you have to do the preparation yourself.

F. Cattabeni   I entirely agree. For TXB_2 and 6-keto-$PGF_{1\alpha}$ there are no suppliers of the deuterated molecules. It would be theoretically possible not to use them. However, since the purification procedure involves many steps, the addition of deuterated internal standards would be of great help. Maybe, the CEE could organize such a service.

N. Poyser   Is it necessary to add inhibitors to rat furdus strip to assay $PGF_{2\alpha}$ if the $PGF_{2\alpha}$ has been purified from a biological sample.

F. Cattabeni   The antagonists of neurotransmitters are added in order to avoid responses due to neurotransmitters present in the organ preparation, I forgot to say that also indomethacin has to be added, in order to prevent local synthesis of PG's.

5 IDENTIFICATION OF PROSTACYCLIN, THROMBOXANE A$_2$ AND PROSTAGLANDINS IN PHARMACOLOGICAL EXPERIMENTS

J.A. Salmon, P. Salzman and S. Moncada

Many authors have determined prostaglandins (PGs) in a novel situation using only one technique, for example bioassay, radioimmunoassay or thin layer chromatography. Data from these experiments may suggest that a PG is produced but the results as to precisely which PG is produced can be misleading. Any conclusion would be more reliable if consistent data is obtained from different types of assay. In this paper we shall describe the experimental design we have used to establish the identity of prostaglandins in pharmacological experiments with particular reference to the recently described identification of prostacyclin and thromboxane A$_2$ in rabbit pulmonary artery (1). We shall attempt to point out some of the pitfalls of using only one type of analytical procedure.

Strips of rabbit intra-pulmonary artery (i.p.a.) exhibit a different pharmacological profile compared with other vascular strips; prostacyclin potently relaxes most other rabbit blood vessels (e.g. coeliac and mesenteric arteries; see 2) but it showed an inconsistent and low activity on i.p.a. Rabbit coeliac and mesenteric artery strips are relaxed by infusions of either arachidonic acid (AA) or the PG endoperoxide, PGH$_2$, which is due to intra-mural conversion to PGI$_2$. However, i.p.a. contracted to both AA and PGH$_2$. The pharmacological responses were not due to conversion of AA (or PGH$_2$) by any tissue other than i.p.a. itself since the i.p.a. had been carefully dissected and thoroughly cleaned of adhering lung tissue, platelets and other blood components (see 1). We decided to explore the mechanism of action of AA (and PGH$_2$) on i.p.a. Our initial approach was to establish whether the response of i.p.a. to AA and PGH$_2$ was a direct effect or due to conversion to active metabolites. This can be conveniently examined by investigating the effect of specific inhibitors of enzymic conversions. Aspirin, indomethacin and meclofenamic acid blocked the response of i.p.a. to AA. Since these drugs inhibit the fatty acid cyclo-oxygenase (3,4) these data indicated that AA was indeed converted by i.p.a. to prostaglandins or thromboxanes.   1-Pentyl-imidazole, an inhibitor of thromboxane synthetase (5) also reduced the response of the tissue to AA which suggested that the biological activity was in part due to formation of thromboxane A_2 (TXA_2).   The response to PGH_2 was different since it was not affected by 1-pentyl imidazole although an enhanced contractile response was observed if the endoperoxide was converted to TXA_2 by horse platelet microsome (HPM) preparation before testing on the bioassay strip. These data suggested that the endoperoxide was not converted by the tissue when applied as a single bolus injection. Both types of inhibitor also lowered the resting tone of i.p.a. suggesting that PGs and TXA_2 contribute to the tone of the tissue (see 1). The use of these specific enzyme inhibitors to indicate the involvement of PGs in biological processes is invaluable.

Often the PGs formed in a perfused organ or tissue can be identified by directing the perfusate over a cascade of superfused assay tissues (6).   The technique gains specificity by careful selection of the assay tissues and by addition of a mixture of antagonists (see 7) to other biologically active components (e.g. adrenaline, 5-HT, histamine). Indomethacin is also added to prevent intra-mural conversion to PGs by the assay tissues. For example, a combination of strips of bovine coronary artery (BCA), rabbit aorta (RbA), rabbit coeliac artery (RbCa), rat stomach (RS) and rat colon (RC) can be used to differentiate between most PGs and thromboxanes (see 2).

In our experiments however, strips of RbA, RbCa and RS did not respond when the fluid superfusing strips of i.p.a. was directed over the above assay tissues even when AA was infused over the i.p.a. These data suggested that, if PGs were indeed formed, the levels were too low to be detected by the assay tissues.

A second type of bioassay which provides useful qualitative data is platelet aggregation; TXA_2 and the PG endoperoxides induce whereas PGI_2, PGE_1 and PGD_2 inhibit aggregation. Incubations of i.p.a. in buffer produced a potent anti-aggregatory compound (Fig 1A); the following data confirmed that the activity was PGI_2:-

1) The activity was almost completely lost during storage at ambient temperature for 30 min whereas it was relatively stable at $0\text{-}4^{\circ}C$ (Fig. 1B).

2) The activity was destroyed by acid but stabilised by alkali.

3) The formation of the inhibitory compound was prevented by prior treatment of i.p.a. with indomethacin or other inhibitors of cyclo-oxygenase.

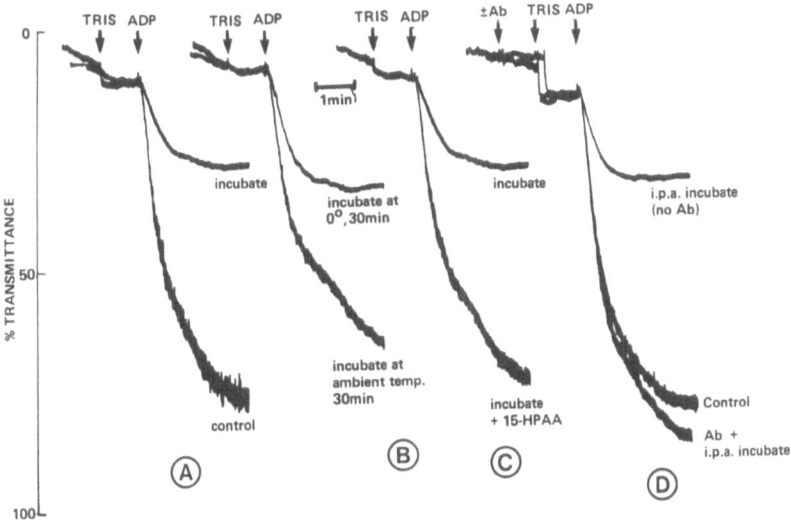

Fig.1 A. *Inhibition of ADP-induced platelet aggregation by rabbit intra-pulmonary artery (i.p.a.) incubated in tris buffer. B. stability of the inhibitory activity at 0°C and ambient temperature; note loss of activity at ambient temperature. C. Inhibition of the formation of the anti-aggregatory activity from i.p.a. by prior incubation of the tissue with 15-hydroperoxy-arachidonic acid (15-HPAA). D. Reduction of the inhibitory activity of i.p.a. by addition of anti-PGI$_1$ serum (Ab) to the platelet-rich plasma.*

These three criteria are probably sufficient for identification of the activity as PGI$_2$ but the following additional tests were performed:

4) The synthesis of the compounds was also inhibited by incubation of the tissue with 15-hydroperoxy-arachidonic acid (15-HPAA; a relatively specific inhibitor of prostacyclin synthetase (8) (Fig. 1C).

5) The anti-aggregatory response was prevented by addition of an antibody directed against 5,6-dihydro-prostacyclin (PGI$_1$) which also effectively binds prostacyclin (9) (Fig. 1D).

Thus, at this stage, we had evidence from the bioassays to suggest that i.p.a. formed PGI$_2$ and TXA$_2$ and possibly other PGs from endogenous substrates and from added arachidonic acid.

In order to establish which PGs could be formed by i.p.a. from exogenous arachidonic acid we performed the following radiochromatographic assays. Rings of i.p.a. were incubated with $1\text{-}[^{14}C\text{-}]$-arachidonic acid for 30 min at $37^{\circ}C$ in tris-HCl buffer (50mM; pH 7.5). The products were extracted by a procedure similar to that described by Frolich (10); initially ice-cold acetone was added to precipitate protein, then neutral lipids in the clear aqueous-acetone layer were removed with hexane and finally the PGs were extracted with chloroform after adjusting the pH of the aqueous phase to 4.0-4.5 with citric acid. The chloroform was removed under nitrogen; the residue was dissolved in chloroform-methanol (2:1 v/v) and this solution was quantitatively applied to a Whatman LKD thin layer chromatography (TLC) plate which was subsequently developed in the organic phase of ethyl acetate, iso-octane, acetic acid and water (110:50:20:100, v/v). The radioactive zones were detected by autoadiography. Two major products were formed which had Rf's identical to authentic 6-keto-PGF$_{1\alpha}$ and TXB$_2$ (0.13 and 0.26 respectively; see Fig. 2) which are the stable degradation products of PGI$_2$ and TXA$_2$

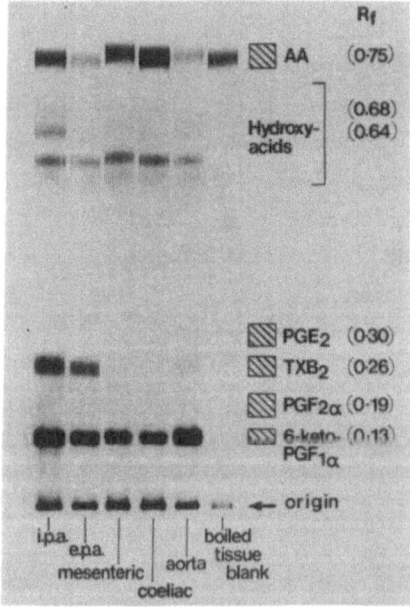

Fig.2 (^{14}C)-Arachidonic acid (AA) conversion by rabbit vasculature (see text for methods). The radioactive zones were detected by auto radiography. Hatched bars indicate the location of standard compounds and the Rf values are in parenthesis.

respectively. It must be emphasised, however, that similarity of Rf in one chromatographic system is insufficient for identification. In fact Cottee et al. (11) showed that 6-keto-PGF$_{1\alpha}$ had an identical Rf to PGE$_2$ or PGF$_{2\alpha}$ in several chromatographic systems. Therefore, the radioactive zones produced by i.p.a. were re-chromatographed in a second solvent system (chloroform, methanol, acetic acid and water; 90:9:1:0.8, v/v) and the presence of 6-keto-PGF$_{1\alpha}$ and TXB$_2$ was again suggested. The ratio of "6-keto-PGF$_{1\alpha}$" to "TXB$_2$" formed was approximately 2. Rings of extra-pulmonary artery (e.p.a.) synthesized similar products although the ratio of "6-keto-PGF$_{1\alpha}$" to "TXB$_2$" was somewhat higher. However, other rabbit vasculature (aorta, coeliac and mesenteric arteries) did not produce "TXB$_2$" (Fig. 2). Pentyl imidazole inhibited production of "TXB$_2$" by i.p.a. and production of both "6-keto-PGF$_{1\alpha}$" and "TXB$_2$" was completely abolished by treatment of i.p.a. with indomethacin. Also, neither radioactive product was detected in boiled tissue control.

Thus, the evidence for the synthesis of TXA$_2$ and PGI$_2$ by i.p.a. was strong. Final proof was obtained by gas-liquid chromatography-mass spectrometry. The "6-keto-PGF$_{1\alpha}$" and "TXB$_2$" zones obtained from replicate incubations of [^{14}C]-AA plus unlabelled AA with i.p.a. were scraped from the TLC plate and the compounds eluted with methanol. After drying off the solvent, the residue was reacted with methoxylamine in pyridine, diazomethane and N,O-bis-(trimethylsilyl)-trifluoroacetamide (BSTFA) with 1% trimethylchlorosilane (TMCS) to form the methoxime, methyl ester and trimethylsilyl ether derivative. Initially, portions of the derivatives in the silylating reagent were injected into a Pye Model 84 gas chromatograph (GC) containing a 1% OV 1 column at 220°C and the effluent was monitored by a flame ionization detector (FID) and a Panax radio-gas chromatograph (RGC) detector. The derivatized "6-keto-PGF$_{1\alpha}$" zone produced a single radioactive GC peak with a retention time (Rt) exactly the same as that of authentic 6-keto-PGF$_{1\alpha}$. However, the "TXB$_2$" zone was resolved into two radioactive GC peaks, one of which had an identical Rt to standard TXB$_2$. Further aliquots of the solutions of the derivatives were injected into a Hewlett-Packard Model 5710 GC combined with a VG Micromass 16F mass spectrometer (MS). The GC conditions were as above and the MS was operated in the electron impact mode at 40eV. The mass spectrum of the derivitized product in the TLC zone at Rf 0.13 confirmed that the compound was 6-keto-PGF$_{1\alpha}$; the spectrum was characterized by major ions at ^{m}/e 378, 418, 508 and 598. Also, one component in the TLC zone of Rf 0.26 was confirmed as TXB$_2$ as the mass spectrum had intense ions at $^m/e$ 211, 301 and 436. The second component in this zone produced a fragmentation pattern with abundant ions at $^m/e$ 310, 375, 425, 465 and 555 which identified it as 13,14-dihydro-6,15-diketo-$PGF_{1\alpha}$. Previously, Wong et al. (12) had identified 6,15-diketo-$PGF_{1\alpha}$ in bovine mesenteric arteries. Both 13,14-dihydro-6,15-diketo-$PGF_{1\alpha}$ and 6,15-diketo-$PGF_{1\alpha}$ are breakdown products of metabolites of prostacyclin. The presence of 13,14-dihydro-6,15-diketo-$PGF_{1\alpha}$ was assumed to explain (i) the faint band of radioactivity at Rf 0.26 produced by samples of aorta (Fig. 2) a tissue which converted more than 30% of added $[^{14}C]$-AA to $[^{14}C]$-6-keto-$PGF_{1\alpha}$ and also (ii) the residual radioactivity recovered as "$[^{14}C]$-TXB_2" after inhibition with 1-pentyl-imidazole. The demonstration that 13,14-dihydro-6,15-diketo-$PGF_{1\alpha}$ had an Rf comparable to TXB_2 further highlights the risk of using TLC mobility as the only criteria for identification of PGs.

Thus the foregoing data demonstrated that PGI_2 and TXA_2 were the major metabolites of AA formed in i.p.a. Further quantitative studies could now confidently be performed using relatively specific radioimmunoassays (RIA) for 6-keto-$PGF_{1\alpha}$ and TXB_2 (13). Firstly, the unstimulated amounts of 6-keto-$PGF_{1\alpha}$ and TXB_2 in i.p.a. were measured by RIA; 0.5-1.0ng 6-keto-$PGF_{1\alpha}$/mg tissue and 100-200pg TXB_2/mg tissue were detected. Secondly, the release of 6-keto-$PGF_{1\alpha}$ and TXB_2 by superfused strips of i.p.a during basal and during infusions of AA could be monitored (see Fig. 3). In these latter experiments, it was clearly shown that both PGI_2 and TXA_2 were produced and that the biological response correlated with the level of thromboxane even though the latter was the minor product. Infusion of 1-pentyl-imidazole greatly decreased the tissue response to AA and also caused a reduction of TXB_2; addition of indomethacin further lowered the tone of the tissue and also inhibited release of 6-keto-$PGF_{1\alpha}$. Thus, the biological response of i.p.a. to AA is primarily mediated by conversion to TXA_2; the remaining part of the contraction is probably due to conversion to PGI_2 but it could also be due to either unconverted PG endoperoxides or degradation products of the endoperoxides (e.g. $PGF_{2\alpha}$) (see ref. 1). Also, the synthesis of TXA_2 and possibly PGI_2 contributes to the resting tone of the tissue. On the other hand, the biological response of the rabbit i.p.a. to single injections of PGH_2 is probably a direct effect since (i) the contraction to PGH_2 is not affected by treatment of the tissue with pentyl-imidazole and (ii) ^{14}C-PGH_2 is not readily metabolized by i.p.a. to either 6-keto $PGF_{1\alpha}$ or TXB_2. Indeed, the main products detected in the superfusion fluid after an injection of ^{14}C-PGH_2 were ^{14}C-PGE_2, $PGF_{2\alpha}$, PGD_2 and HHT.

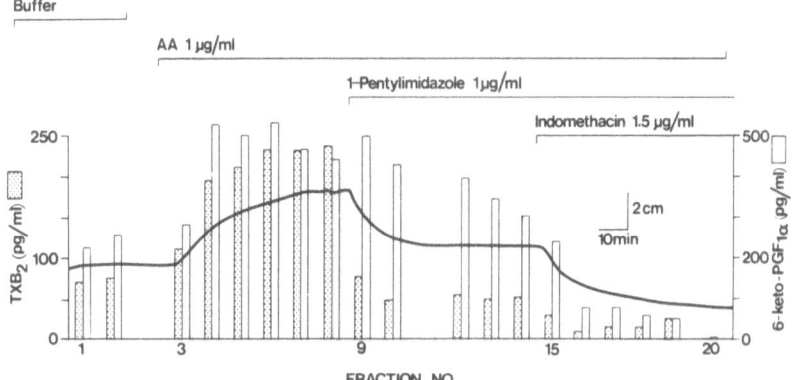

Fig.3 Release of arachidonic acid (AA) metabolites during AA superfusion of rabbit intra-pulmonary artery (i.p.a.) strips. The effluent from 4 i.p.a. strips was analysed for 6-keto-PGF$_{1\alpha}$ (pg/ml; open bars) and TBX$_2$ (pg/ml; stippled bars) by radio-immunoassay in consecutive 10 min fractions. The biological response of i.p.a. during this time is indicated by the overlying heavy line. Buffer only, AA, 1-pentyl-imidazole and indomethacin were applied at the indicated final concentrations during the periods denoted by the horizontal lines. Time scales are the same for tissue response and bar graph.

In conclusion, thromboxane A$_2$ and PGI$_2$ are both synthesized by rabbit intra-pulmonary artery and this probably explains its unusual pharmacological response to arachidonic acid. If these in vitro observations reflect the behaviour of the pulmonary circulation in vivo, then the production of TXA$_2$ by lung vasculature and the response of the pulmonary blood vessels to TXA$_2$ and PGI$_2$ could explain the susceptability of rabbits (even after treatment with anti-platelet serum) to infusions of arachidonic acid (14,15,16). This study serves to illustrate the advantage of using a combination of analytical techniques; the use of only one of the procedures could have produced misleading if not inaccurate data. We consider that the use of at least two different assay procedures is essential for confident identification of prostaglandins and related compounds in biological situations.

References

1. Salzman PM, Salmon JA and Moncada S: Prostacyclin and thromboxane
    A$_2$ synthesis by rabbit pulmonary artery. Submitted for publication,
    1980.

2. Moncada S, Ferreira SH, Vane JR: Bioassay of prostaglandins and
    biologically active substances derived from arachidonic acid. In:
    Advances in prostaglandin and thromboxane research, Vol. 5. Frölich JC
    (ed). New York, Raven Press, 1978, p 211-236.

3. Vane JR: Inhibition of prostaglandin synthesis as a mechanism of action
    for aspirin-like drugs. Nature (Lond.) (231):232-235, 1971.

4. Flower RJ: Drugs which inhibit prostaglandin biosynthesis. Pharmacol.
    Rev. (26):33-67, 1974.

5. Tai HH, Yuan B: On the inhibitory potency of imidazole and its
    derivatives on thromboxane synthetase. Biochem. Biophys. Res.
    Commun. (80):236-242, 1978.

6. Vane JR: The use of isolated organs for detecting active substances in
    the circulating blood. Brit. J. Pharmacol. Chemother. (23):360-373,
    1964.

7. Gilmore N, Vane JR, Wyllie JH: Prostaglandins released by the spleen.
    Nature (Lond.) (218):1135-1140, 1968.

8. Moncada S, Gryglewski RJ, Bunting S, Vane JR: A lipid peroxide inhibits
    the enzyme in blood vessel microsomes that generates from
    prostaglandin endoperoxides the substance (prostaglandin X) which
    prevents platelet aggregation. Prostaglandins (12):715-737, 1976.

9. Bunting S, Moncada S, Reed P, Salmon JA, Vane JR: An antiserum to
    5,6-dihydro-prostacyclin (PGI$_1$) which also binds prostacyclin.
    Prostaglandins (15):565-573.

10. Frölich JC: Gas chromatography - mass spectrometry of prostaglandins.
    In: The Prostaglandins, Vol. 3. Ramwell, PW (ed). New York, Plenum
    Press, 1976, p 1-39.

11. Cottee F, Flower RJ, Moncada S, Salmon JA, Vane JR: Synthesis of 6-
    koto PCF$_{1\alpha}$ by ram seminal vesicle microsomes. Prostaglandins
    (14):413-423, 1977.

12. Wong PY-K, Sun FF, McGiff JC: Metabolism of prostacyclin in blood
    vessels. J. Biol. Chem. (253):5555-5557, 1978.

13. Salmon JA: A radioimmunoassay for 6-keto-prostaglandin F$_{1\alpha}$.
    Prostaglandins (15):383-397, 1978.

14. Amezcua JL, Parsons M, Moncada A: Unstable metabolites of
    arachidonic acid. Aspirin and the formation of the haemostatic plug.
    Throm. Res. (13):477-488, 1978.

15. Bayer BL, Blass KE, Forster W: Anti-aggregatory effect of prostacyclin (PGI$_2$) in vivo. Brit. J. Pharmacol. (66):10-12, 1979.

16. Silver M, Hock W, Kocsis J, Ingerman C, Smith B: Arachidonic acid causes sudden death in rabbits. Science (183):1085-1087, 1974.

6 ANALYSIS OF PROSTANOIDS AND THEIR METABOLITES BY GAS CHROMATOGRAPHY-MASS SPECTROMETRY

C. Fischer, B. Rosenkranz and J.C. Frölich

1. INTRODUCTION

The late discovery and evaluation of prostanoids can be explained in part by the special methods which are required for the isolation and detection of this class of compounds (1-7). Significant progress in biomedical research is often coupled to the development of methods useful for the assay of the compound of interest. In the case of prostanoids the investigator is confronted with a number of difficulties. These include the requirement for a very high degree of specificity of analysis because in addition to the compounds of interest many closely related compounds are present in biological fluids. For example, human urine contains in addition to PGE_2 a large number of PGE_2-metabolites, one of which is present in 10-fold higher concentrations than the parent compound. In plasma, levels of the circulating metabolite of $PGF_{2\alpha}$, 15-keto-13,14-dihydro-$PGF_{2\alpha}$, are 10 to 70-fold higher than those of $PGF_{2\alpha}$. Furthermore, prostanoids bind with high affinity to their receptors and sometimes non-specifically to proteins. The high affinity, low capacity specific binding implies that low concentrations are already biologically relevant. Estimation of prostanoid blood levels based on excretion rates of major metabolites in the urine determined by gas chromatography-mass spectrometry (GC/MS) and plasma half-life determination indicate levels of $PGF_{2\alpha}$ of less than 3 pg/ml and of PGE_2 of less than 14 pg/ml (8). It can be seen that assays of extreme sensitivity are necessary to measure these values. Problems also arise when collecting a biological sample. In blood, platelets rapidly activate phospholipase and form cyclic endoperoxides which can be converted to PGE_2, $PGF_{2\alpha}$ and TXA_2 and lead to falsely high blood levels. In tissues, excision and ischemia provide powerful stimuli to prostaglandin synthesis. For these reasons measurement of circulating levels of the primary prostaglandins has been largely abandoned and metabolites are measured instead. Finally, prostanoids are chemically labile substances and can be converted into other prostanoids by dehydration and isomerization (9, 10). The detection system has to fullfill two requirements: specificity and sensitivity. The GC/MS methods pioneered by Samuelsson, Hamberg (11-15) and Axen (16, 17) have met these requirements. These researchers developed the idea of the use of a deuterated analog of the prostanoid for the purposes of internal standard and carrier. The deuterated prostanoid is added in known quantity to a biological sample and the ratio of it to the endogenous prostanoid determined with the help of the mass spectrometer. This method has yielded the most reliable data to date. Its applicability to all prostanoids and their metabolites gives it a broad range of applications. It has been shown to be of particular value in human investigation where other methods often have failed (see for example comparison of GC/MS data and radioimmunoassay data in the paper of Gill et al. (18)).

Other methods applied to the measurement of prostanoids include gas chromatography with electron capture detection (19-21), bioassay (22), competitive receptor binding assays (23) and radioimmunoassays (24). It is important to check these assays against GC/MS which is considered the reference method.

In the last few years the GC/MS technique was improved by the use of high pressure liquid chromatography (HPLC) for sample work up (25) and by capillary gas chromatographic columns (21, 26). We would like to report about some of these improvements.

2. EXTRACTION AND PURIFICATION PROCEDURES

To introduce samples into the GC/MS-system several purification steps are needed. Subsequently, volatile derivatives must be synthesized before the sample can be injected into the gas chromatograph. Some details will be discussed.

There are different ways for extraction depending on the biological material - fluid or tissue - and on the prostanoid. A deuterium labeled internal standard is added before extraction. Syntheses of these internal standards has been described (14, 27). They are applied in excess over the expected biological level to reduce the absorption of the endogenous prostanoid and minimize the losses of sample. In addition, a negligible amount of tritiated compound with high specific activity is added to the sample and indicates the course of sample preparation. This tracer allows to calculate the recoveries for the different purification steps by liquid scintillation counting of the chromatographic effluents. Some extraction methods have been described recently (27-29). Chloroform is polar enough for an extraction of PGE_2 and $PGF_{2\alpha}$ with more than 90 % from the aqueous phase. For the more polar prostanoid 6-keto-$PGF_{1\alpha}$ an efficient extraction can be achieved only with ethylacetate.

The application of short open columns to remove proteins and electrolytes and to achieve group separation are discussed in several papers and reviews (27-29).

2.1 SEPARATION BY HIGH PRESSURE LIQUID CHROMATOGRAPHY (HPLC)

The problem of selective separation could be solved by the introduction of high pressure liquid chromatography with its many advantages (25, 29-31):

1. separation of closely related compounds
2. mild conditions
3. good recoveries (about 80-90 %)
4. excellent reproducibility
5. small elution volumes of 2-3 ml for each peak
6. use of the column for several 100 times

7. flexibility in programming of the solvent mixtures.

High pressure liquid chromatography affords accuracy and specificity. Retention volumes help in identification as they are reliable in a conditioned HPLC-system.

Nevertheless one should have in mind that more than one compound can be under one peak. In one of the chromatografic systems described (28) PGE_2, 6K-$PGF_{1\alpha}$ and TXB_2 are eluted together. The subsequent application of a reversed phase column provides their resolution (28). The HPLC is very flexible as several parameters can be changed:

1. the type of column-silica, straight phase or reversed phase (chemically bonded alkyl and/or aryl groups on silica surface). For reversed phase applications we found the "fatty acid column" (Waters Assoc.) particularly useful (29)

2. the mixture of solvents (2 or 3)

3. the composition of the solvent mixture as a function of time.

After our introduction of HPLC for the purification of biological samples for GC/MS and other applications (25) we have been able to apply it to a large number of separation problems. Currently, we are using HPLC for the purification of PGE_2, $PGF_{2\alpha}$, 15-keto-dihydro-$PGF_{2\alpha}$, 6-keto-$PGF_{1\alpha}$, 7α-hydroxi, 5,11 diketo-tetranorprosta–1,16-dioic acid, and for the separation of polar metabolites of 6-keto-$PGF_{1\alpha}$ and PGI_2 (29, 32).

Other clean-up operations without use of HPLC can lead to an adequate purification applicable for GC/MS-measurement (33).

Besides, the application of thin-layer chromatography can be sufficient depending on the biological sample and the prostanoids which are to be analyzed (28).

2.2 GAS-CHROMATOGRAPHY

2.2.1 Derivatization

Prostanoids have several functional groups namely carboxyl-, hydroxi-and carbonylgroups. For GC-application the derivatization of these reactive groups is necessary to generate volatile and thermostabile compounds.

In most cases the carboxylgroup is derivatized to the methylester by treatment with diazomethane, the ketogroups to the methoximes by treatment with methoxiamine. HCl, the hydroxigroups to the trimethylsilylethers by silylating reagents as N,O-bis (trimethylsilyl)-trifluoracetamid (BSTFA), N,O-bis(trimethylsilyl)-acetamid (BSA) or N-trimethylsilylimidazol (TSIM) with or without a base such as pyridine.

Some investigators prefer to inject the prostanoids with the free keto-function. An assay for PGE_2 has been described where the purified extract with PGE_2-methylester is transformed to PGE_2-methylester-trimethylsilylester by treatment with BSTFA (34).

Some important requirements for a derivatization reaction for GC/MS-use are listed:

1. It must be quantitative.
2. It must lead to one definite product.
3. It must be suitable for GC-conditions:
    volatile, thermostabile, no or little absorption on the column filling material.
4. It must result in a compound with an ionization pattern of high fragments for a specific measurement in selected ion monitoring (SIM)-mode.

For many prostanoids suitable derivates for a GC/MS-determination are known. Nevertheless, attempts are still fruitful to synthesize better compounds which are more stable against hydrolysis and offer a simpler fragmentation pattern.

Higher m/z-values in general offer the advantage of lower chance of interfering from other compounds. Different silylating reagents as dimethylethyl-imidazol, dimethyl-propylimidazol (35) or dimethyltertiary butyl-chlorsilan (36) result in compounds with a high molecular weight and often a very simple fragmentation. The applications of these reagents is described only in a few papers. It would be interesting to know their usefulness for prostanoid derivatization for quantitative analysis.

Other stable derivates are the butylboronates with their advantage of very low absorption on the GC-column. In this way the amount of internal standard can be reduced as no carrier effect is needed (37). The reaction with butylboronic acid is limited to prostanoids with two hydroxigroups in the pentane ring.

We have recently reported on a new derivative for the analysis of PGE_2 which has the following advantages over the derivate PGE_2-methylester-methoxime-trimethylsilylether (PGE_2-Me-MOX-TMS_2) used so far. In contrast to PGE_2-Me-MOX-TMS_2 which exists in two isomeres this derivate is a single chemical identity. It has better gas chromatographic properties and shows a very suitable fragmentation pattern which allows measurement of as low as 1 ng injected into a glass capillary column without use of carrier (38).

2.2.2 Packed and glass capillary columns

During the last years glass capillary columns have replaced packed columns in many laboratories. The packed column has limited resolution and therefore less specifity. Many investigators routinely now work with commercially available capillary columns.

Excellent separations have been demonstrated with self prepared capillary columns (26). The comparison between packed columns and glass capillary columns revealed a 100 fold improvement in sensitivity of the glass capillary column measured with flame ionisation detector (26).

The problem of adsorption on the surface of columns which reduce the efficiency of packed columns as well as glass capillary column will probably be solved by new flexible fused silica columns. This column material (amorphous silica) gives a neutral character to the column surface. So with this column inertness the difficulties with adsorption of small amounts of sample will probably be reduced.

We had an analytical problem because of the discrepancy in the ratio of two ion pairs used for the SIM-mode quantification of $PGF_{2\alpha}$. The ratio of the ion pairs with m/z 423.3 and 513.3 for the endogenous $PGF_{2\alpha}$ and with m/z 427.3 and 517.3 for the internal standard, the 3, 3, 4, 4-^{2}H-deuterated $PGF_{2\alpha}$, were calculated by the peak areas. The tracings for the endogenous $PGF_{2\alpha}$ revealed interfering peaks, see Figure 1A, which make the proper measurement impossible. Therefore, we changed the parameters of the temperature program. In contrast to the first injection the peaks of the second run had longer retention times which leads to a separation from the interfering peaks, see Figure 1B. The quantification was now possible. The ion ratios were 0.034 for the upper ion pair and 0.032 for the lower ion pair with a mean of 0.033. The blank was determined by injecting the internal standard by itself. In the channel for the non-deuterated $PGF_{2\alpha}$ a peak appeared corresponding to 0.003 of the peak in the tracing of the deuterated tracing. The calculation reveals that the sample contains 700 ng x 0.033 = 23.01 ng. The blank (700 ng x 0.003 = 0.21) needs to be subtracted (23.01 ng - 0.21 ng) and yields as final result 22.9 ng. Since 1/30th of a 24 hour urine was used, the total amount of $PGF_{2\alpha}$ excreted was 687 ng/24 h.

3. Mass spectrometry

3.1 Quality control

Assays in SIM-mode and EI-technique exist for many prostanoids and in principle can be set up for all prostanoids and their metabolites. The well equipped mass spectrometers - in most cases quadrupole mass spectrometers - are easy to operate. For quantification of prostanoids the selected-ion-monitoring in electron inpact mode reveals excellent specifity and sensitivity (27). The responses of selected pairs of ions of high relative abundance are compared. As the amount of added deuterated internal standard is known the ratios of the endogenous prostanoid signal and the one of the internal standard allow quantification (27).

If the synthesized derivatives reveal ionization with high fragments and these are produced in high relative abundance a sensitive and specific measurement can be achieved.

To make sure that the peaks detected by GC/MS correspond to the wanted prostanoid some parameters can be varied as the length and kind of the GC-column, the temperature program and the monitored ions. If the peak ratios of various ion pairs remain constant a high degree of reliability for the measurement has been achieved.

With the radioimmunoassay only the counts of radioactivity serve as basis for quanitification (24). In this way diverse results were obtained and interpretations often are contractictory. Efforts are made to improve the antibodies, and now some radioimmunoassays exist which deliver levels with good correspondence to levels obtained by GC/MS-measurement.

Different parameters of the GC/MS-measurement in SIM-mode quantification permit a critical examination of the tracings. The gas chromatographic parameters as peak shape, shoulders, interfering peaks, drifting of the base-line and the retention time allow judgement which of the peaks can reasonably be taken for the calculation. Concerning the mass spectrometric datas we recommend the use of at least two ion pairs for the quantification of any prostanoid in SIM-mode. The comparison of the ion pair ratios serves as a control for specific measurement. We use as a routine check not only comparison of the ion ratios of the deuterated and non-deuterated ion pair but also the ratio of the two different deuterated and non-deuterated ions, i.e. the ratio of 517.3 to 427.3 and the ratio of 513.3 to 423.3 of Fig. 1. These latter ratios can be obtained from mass spectra of the pure compounds and are not dependent on the amount of prostanoid in the biological sample.

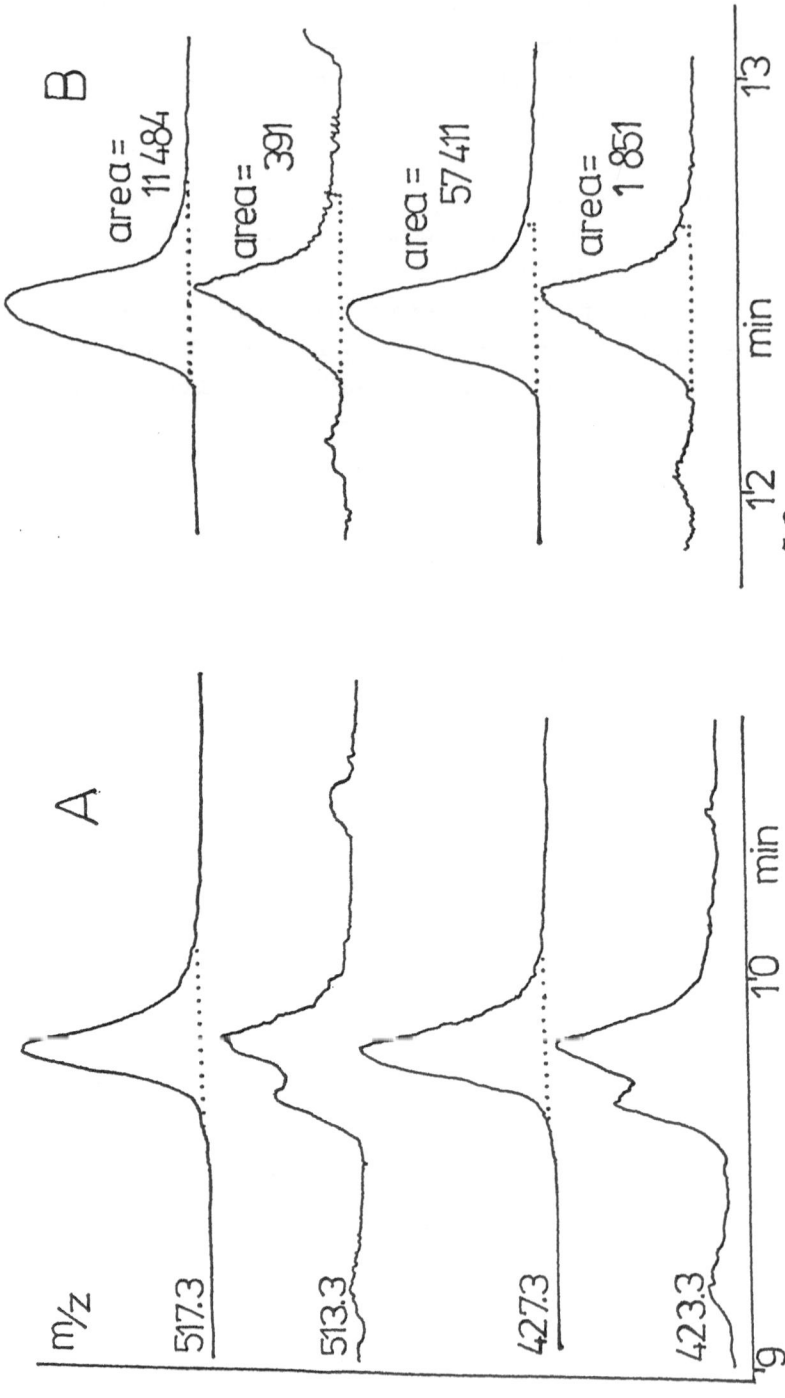

Fig. 1: Measurement of PGF$_{2\alpha}$ in human urine by SIM-mode with 3, 3, 4, 4-[^{2}H$_4$]-PGF$_{2\alpha}$ as internal standard. A: Injection of a 70 ml extraction sample with multistep temperature program. B: Injection of the same sample with a prolonged retention time due to different temperature program.

3.2 Ionization mode

Chemical ionization (CI) mass spectrometry can be applied to structural elucidation and quantitative determinations. Several publications report about successful determinations (39, 40). R.W. Walker et al. (41) describe an assay for the major metabolite in man of prostaglandin E_1 and E_2 by CI. After elution from a packed GC-column the samples were detected by mass-spectrometry with methane as reagent gas. The energy involved in the processes of CI mass spectrometry is low compared to EI-mode and depends upon the reactand gas used (methane, isomethane, ammonia). This low energy often leads to an enhancement in the abundance of ions formed in the molecular ion region. This effect is wellcome as the higher the m/z values used for SIM-mode the more specific is the quantification. GC/MS measurement in the CI-technique seems to be a promising alternative to EI-technique, even though little information on its use in quantitative analysis of prostanoids has come to light.

3.3 Computer control of data analysis

Computers have assumed an important role in analysis of data acquired by mass spectrometry. Mass spectrometric data are particulary suited for coupling to computers because all of their functions can be readily controlled by a computer and because the mass spectrometer generates a large number of data points. For example, the GC/MS run shown in Fig. 2 required storage and analysis of at least 250 000 data points.

Fig. 2 (see next page)

Analysis of urinary metabolite of 6-keto-PGF$_{1\alpha}$. A: Total ion current tracing of peak obtained by HPLC from urine following infusion of radioactive 6-keto-PGF$_{1\alpha}$. 329 scans in the mass range m/z 300–700 were recorded. From the total ion current no identification of a metabolite was possible. The HPLC behaviour of the metabolite made it likely that it was dinor-6keto-PGF$_{1\alpha}$. Therefore a reconstructed ion chromatogram for prominent ions of this metabolite i.e. m/z 570, 480 and 350 was obtained from the computer data file. B: shows which peak of the total ion current represents this metabolite. Instrument: HP 5985 A.

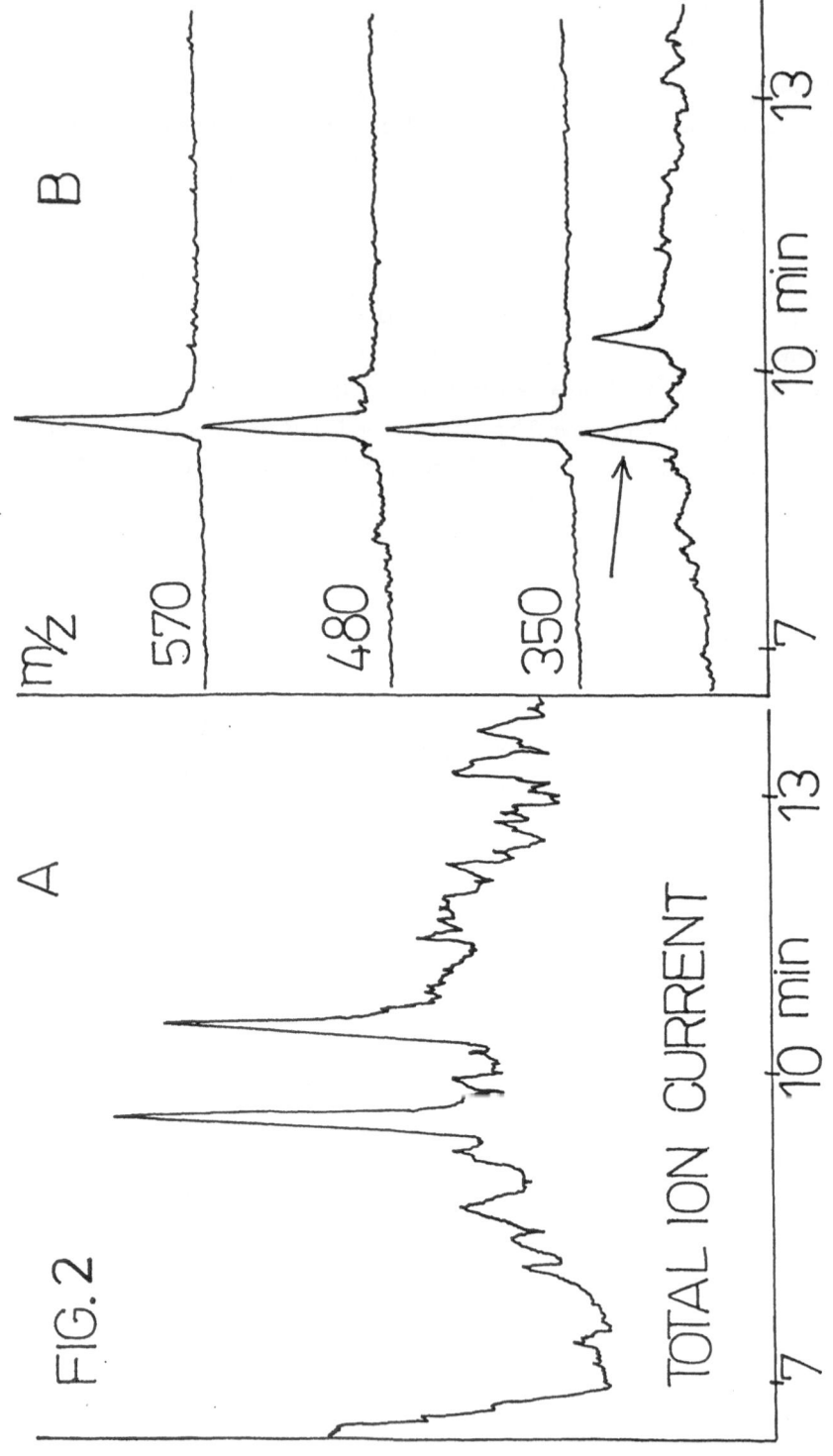

FIG. 2

A

B

TOTAL ION CURRENT

m/z

570

480

350

7   10 min   13

7   10 min   13

While in the SIM-mode less sophisticated devices have shown to be quite satisfactory computers are particulary useful in the identification of unknown compounds. We would like to present an example from our work on metabolism of PGI_2 in man after infusion of deuterated, tritiated and unlabeled PGI_2 (32). Extraction and HPLC-separation were carried out.

After injection of one of the HPLC-peaks into the GC/MS two big and several small peaks appeared in the total ion current, a tracing that has some similarity to a flame ionization detector of a GC. During the run of seven minutes 329 scans were acquired in the mass range of m/z 300 - 700. An analysis of these scans was made by reconstructed ion chromatograms which revealed that the spectrum number 129 with the prominent ions 570,480 and 350 m/z can be assigned to the metabolite dinor-6keto-$PGF_{1\alpha}$. Plotting the mass spectrum of this scan number 129 confirms the identity of this metabolite with dinor-6keto-$PGF_{1\alpha}$.

Mass spectra of biological samples are often accompanied by a considerable amount of background, see Fig. 3 A. Therefore, we wanted a substraction of nonspecific traces. This chore used to be done by hand, a tedious and less-than-inspiring task. With the help of the computer system background subtraction can easely performed, see Fig. 3 B.

The computer owns the capacity for controlling the GC/MS-functions and for storage large numbers of data points. Programs like reconstructed ion chromatogram, background subtraction, comparison and subtraction of different sample runs help and facilitate the evaluation of the acquisitated data and identification of unknown compounds.

Fig. 3 (see next page):

Mass spectrum of 6-keto-$PGF_{1\alpha}$ derivatized as methylester-methoxime-trimethylsilylether, obtained by HPLC from urine following infusion of radioactive 6-keto-$PGF_{1\alpha}$ and injected into the GC/MS.

A: Scan number 199 from the total of 331 scans acquired in the mass range from m/z 300-700.

B. The same scan number after background subtraction by aid of a computer program. In this case, scan number 179 was substracted from scan 199.

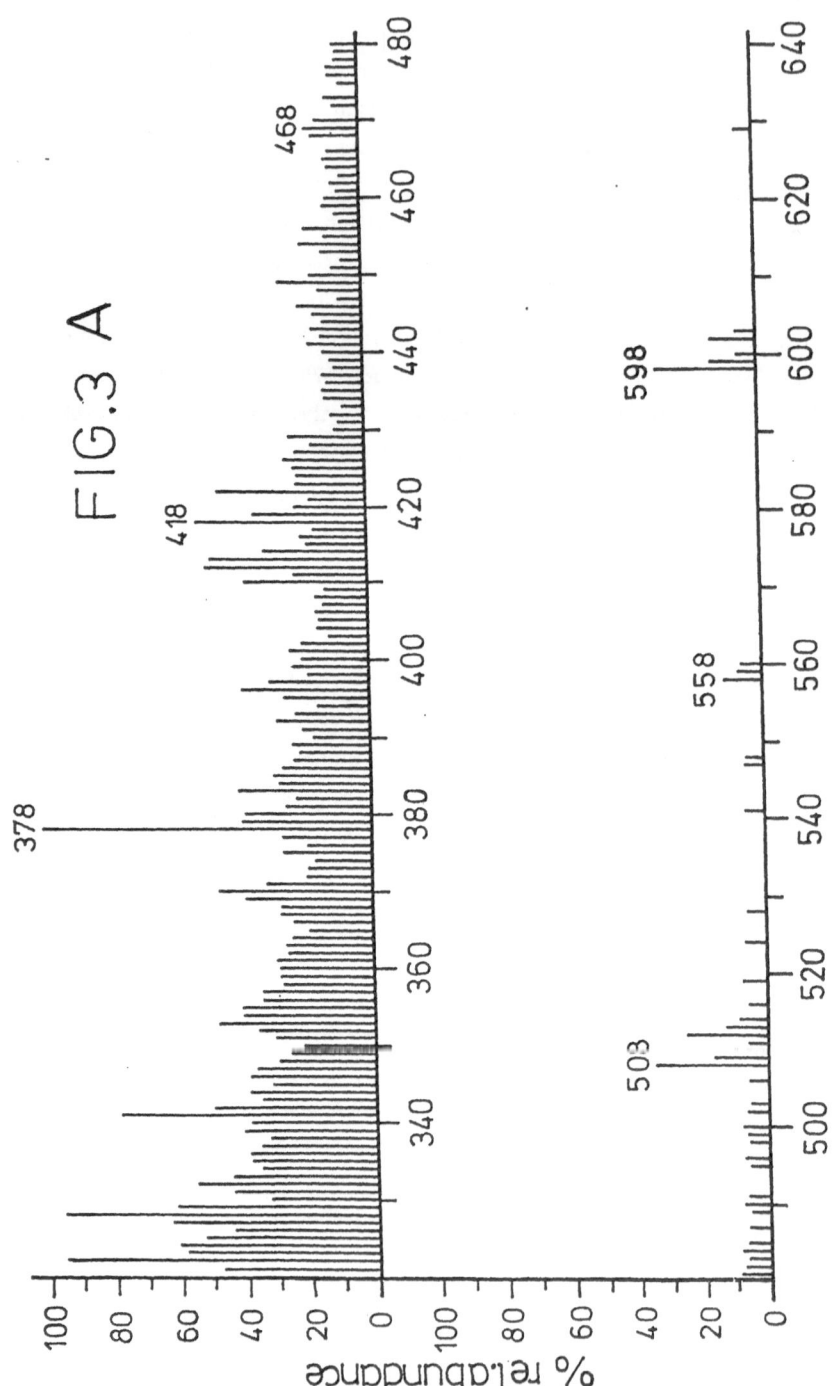

FIG.3 A

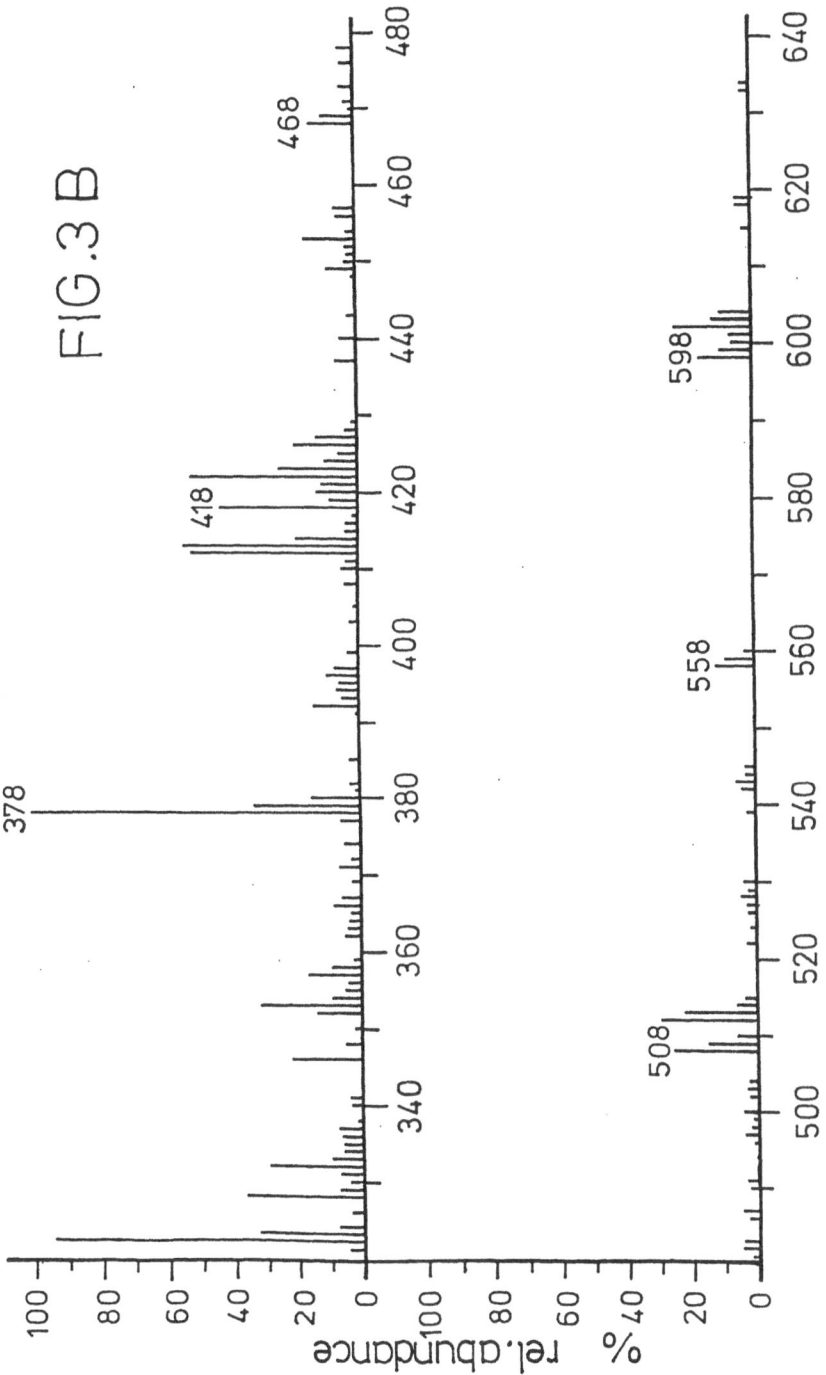

FIG.3 B

References

1. Goldblatt, M.W.: A depressor substance in seminal fluid. J. Soc. Chem. Ind. (London) 52:1056-1057, 1933

2. von Euler, U.S.: Zur Kenntnis der pharmakologischen Wirkungen von Nativesekreten und Extrakten männlicher accessorischer Geschlechtsdrüsen. Arch. Exp. Pathol. Pharmakol. (Naunyn-Schmiedebergs) 175:78-84, 1934

3. von Euler, U.S.: Die spezifische blutdrucksenkende Substanz in der menschlichen Prostata und in Samenvesikelsekretionen. Klin. Wochenschrift 14:1182-1183, 1935

4. Bergström, S., Sjövall, J.: The isolation of prostaglandin F from sheep prostate glands. Acta Chem. Scand. 14:1693-1701, 1960

5. Bergström, S., Ryhage, R., Samuelsson, B., Sjövall, J.: The structures of prostaglandin E_1, F_1 and F1ß. J. Biol. Chem. 238:3555-3564, 1963

6. Bergström, S., Dressler, F., Ryhage, R., Samuelsson, B., Sjövall, J.: The isolation of two further prostaglandins from sheep prostate glands. Ark. Kemi 19:563-567, 1962

7. Samuelsson, B.: The structure of prostaglandin E_3. J. Am. Chem. Soc. 85:1878-1879, 1963

8. Frölich, J.C., McGiff, J.C., Needleman, P., Gill, J.R., Nies, A.S.: Report of the hypertension task force. Vol. 7, Prostaglandins. US-DHEW-NIH Publication No. 79-1629, Washington, DC, 1979, pp.1-101

9. Monkhouse, D.C., van Campen, L. and Aguiar, A.J.: Kinetics of dehydration and isomerization of prostaglandin E_1 and E_2. J. Pharm. Sci. 62:576-580, 1973

10. Frölich, J.C., Sweetman, B.J., Carr, K. and Oates, J.A.: Prostaglandin synthesis in rabbit renal medulla. Life Sci. 17:1105-1112, 1975

11. Hamberg, M., Svensson, J., and Samuelsson, B.: Prostaglandin endoperoxides. A new concept concerning the mode of action and release of prostaglandins. Proc. Natl. Acad. Sci. 71:3824-3828, 1974

12. Hamberg, M.: Inhibition of prostaglandin synthesis in man. Biochem. Biophys. Res. Commun. 49:720-726, 1972

13. Hamberg, M.: Quantitative studies on prostaglandin synthesis in man -II- Determinations of the major metabolite of prostaglandins $F_{1\alpha}$ and $F_{2\alpha}$. Anal. Biochem. 55:365-378, 1973

14. Axen, U., Gréen, K., Hörlin, D. and Samuelsson, B.: Mass spectrometric determination of picomole amounts of prostaglandins E_2 and $F_{2\alpha}$ using synthetic deuterium labeled carriers. Biochem. Biophys. Res. Commun. 45:519-525, 1971

15. Gréen, K., Granström, E., Samuelsson, B. and Axen, U.: Methods for quantitative analysis of $PGF_{2\alpha}$, PGE_2, 9α, 11α, 15-keto-prost-5-enoic acid and 9α, 11α, 15-trihydroxy-prost-5-enoic acid from body fluids using deuterated carriers and gas chromatography-mass spectrometry. Anal. Biochem. 54:434-453, 1973

16. Axen, U.: Synthetic approaches to prostaglandins in: Annual Reports in Medicinal chemistry 1967, CK Cain, Academic Press, N.Y.:290-296, 1969

17. Axen, U., Baczynskyj, L., Duchamp, D., Zieserl, J.: Gaschromatography-mass spectrometry assay for prostaglandins, J. Reprod. Med. 9:372-375, 1972

18. Gill, J.R., Frölich, J.C., Bowden, R.E., Taylor, A.A., Keiser, H.R., Seyberth, H.W., Oates, J.A., Bartter, F.C.: Bartters Syndrome: A disorder characterized by high urinary prostaglandins and a dependence of hyperreninemia on prostaglandin synthesis. Am. J. Med. 61:43-51, 1976

19. Jouvenaz, G., Nugteren, D., Beerthuis, R. and van Dorp, D.: A sensitive method for the determination of prostaglandins by gaschromatography with electron-capture detection. Biochim. Biophys. Acta 202:232-234, 1970

20. Fitzpatrick, F.A.: Gas chromatography of the prostaglandins in: Advances in Prostaglandin and Thromboxane Research, J.C. Frölich ed., Vol. 5:95-118,1978

21. Fitzpatrick, F.A., Stringfellow, D.A., Maclouf, J. and Rigaud, M.: Glass capillary gas chromatography with electron capture detection. Separation of Prostaglandins. J. Chrom. 177:51-60, 1979

22. Moncada, S., Ferreira, S.H., Vane, J.R.: Advances in Prostaglandin and Thromboxane Research, Vol. 5 (J.C. Frölich, ed.,):211-236, 1978

23. Frölich, J.C., Williams, W.M., Sweetman, B.J., Smigel, M., Carr, K., Hollifield, J.W., Fleischer, S., Nies, A.S., Frisk-Holmberg and Oates, J.A.: Analysis of renal prostaglandin synthesis by competitive protein binding assay and gas chromatography -mass spectrometry. Adv. in Prostaglandin and Thromboxane Research Vol. 1 (D. Samuelsson, R. Paoletti, ed.):65-80, 1976

24. Granström, E. and Kindahl, H.: Radioimmunoassay of prostaglandins and thromboxanes. Adv. in Prostaglandin and Thromboxane Research Vol. 5 (J.C. Frölich, ed.): 119-210, 1978

25. Carr, K., Sweetman, B.J., Frölich, J.C.: High performance liquid chromatography of prostaglandins, Prostaglandins 11:3-14, 1976

26. Maclouf, J., Rigaud, M., Durand, J. and Chebroux, P.: Glass capillary columns applied to prostaglandins measurement: a useful tool for gas chromatography mass spectrometry analysis. Prostaglandins 11(6):999-1017, 1976

27. Gréen, K., Hamberg, M., Samuelsson, B. and Frölich, J.C.: Measurement of prostaglandins, thromboxanes, prostacyclin and their metabolites by gas - liquid chromatography - mass spectrometry. Adv. in Prostaglandin and Thromboxane Research Vol. 5(J.C.Frölich, ed.):38-94, 1978

28. Gréen, K., Hamberg, M., Samuelsson, B. and Frölich, J.C.: Extraction and chromatographic procedures for purification of prostaglandins, thromboxanes, prostacyclin and their metabolites. Adv. in Prostaglandin and Thromboxane Research Vol. 5 (J.C.Frölich, ed.):15-38, 1978

29. Frölich, J.C.: Gas - chromatography - mass spectrometry of prostaglandins. The Prostaglandins, Vol. 3:1-39, 1977

30. Dunham, E. and Anders, M.: High speed liquid chromatographic analysis of prostaglandins in rat kidney.
Prostaglandins 4:85-92, 1973

31. Anderson, N.H. and Leavey, A.M.K.: Identification and quantitative determination of prostaglandins by high pressure liquid chromatography. Prostaglandins 6:361-374, 1974

32. Rosenkranz, B., Fischer, C., Reimann, I., Weimer, K.E., Beck, G., Frölich, J.C.: Identification of the major metabolite of prostacyclin and 6-keto-prostaglandin $F_{1\alpha}$ in man. Biochim. Biophys. Acta. in press

33. Ferretti, A. and Flanagan, V.P.: A simple, selected ion monitoring method for the determination of prostaglandins E_2 and $F_{2\alpha}$ in human urine. Biomed. Mass Spectr. 6(10):431-434, 1979

34. Lagarde, M., Dechavanne, M., Rigaud, M., Durand, J.: Basal level of human platelet prostaglandins: PGE_1 is more elevated than PGE_2. Prostaglandins 17:685-701, 1979

35. Miyzahi, H., Ishibashi, M. , Yamashita, K. and Katori, M.: Use of new silylating agents for separation and identification of prostaglandins by gas chromatography and gas chromatography - mass spectrometry. J. Chrom. 153:83-90, 1978

36. Brash, A.R., Baillie, Th., A.: A comparison of t-butyl-dimethylsilyl- and trimethylsilyl ether derivates for the characterization of urinary metabolites of prostaglandin $F_{2\alpha}$ by gas chromatography mass spectrometry. Biomed. Mass Spectr. 5(5):346-356, 1978

37. Kelly, R.W.: Method for the measurement of prostaglandin $F_{2\alpha}$ in biological fluids by gas chromatography - mass spectrometry. Anal. Chem. 45(12):2079-2081, 1973

38. Fischer, C.: A new derivate for GC/MS-measurement of prostaglandin E_2. Naunyn-Schmiedeberg's Archives of Pharmacology Supplement to Vol. 311, R29, 1980

39. Osswald, E.O.: Parks, D., Eling, T., Corbett, B.J.: Characterization of prostaglandins by chemical ionization mass spectrometry. J. Chrom. 93:47-62, 1974

40. Ariga, T., Suzuki, M., Morita, I., Murota, S.-J. and Miyatake, T.: Chemical ionization mass spectrometry of trimethylsilyl derivatives of various prostaglandins. Anal. Biochem. 30:174-182, 1978

41. Walker, R.W., Gruber, V.F., Pile, J., Yabumoto, K., Rosegay, A., Taub, D., L'E.Dome, M., Wolf, F.J. and Vandenheuvel, W.J.A.: Capillary column gas - liquid chromatographic mass spectrometric assay for 7α-hydroxy-5,11-diketotetranorprostane 1,16-dioic acid, the major human urinary metabolite of prostaglandins E_1 and E_2. J.Chrom. 181:85-89, 1980

ACKNOWLEDGEMENTS

The internal standards used in these studies were kindly provided by Dr. U. Axen (Upjohn, Kalamazoo, Mich., U.S.A.).

This work was supported by the Robert Bosch Foundation, Stuttgart, Germany (FRG).

DISCUSSION

M. Claeys   1. Concerning the method : do you have any idea about the detection limit for measurement in urine?

2. How do you make the standard curve, to be more specific, how do you prepare the standards used to make the standard curve ?

H. Seyberth   1. Detection limit in biological samples (urine) is between 100 to 200 ng per injection.

2. We just derivatized the standard solution to see the principle detection limit of the instruments and to see the linearity of the standard curve.

J. Frölich   Dr. Seyberth you are showing a patient with Bartter Syndrome of whom you claim that he has normal urinary PGE_2-levels. I would like to challenge this view. In our experience we have found that all patients with this syndrome have elevated urinary PGE_2 levels (1).All of our patients showed the typical signs and symptoms of the syndrome and were untreated at the time of study. Certainly, a number of factors can have influence on urinary prostaglandin levels and we have shown angiotensin II (2) and ADH (3) to be among them. In addition I would like to question your interpretation of your data. It is true that the 24-hour excretion of PGE_2 of your patient is not different from your normal controls. However, when your data are expressed as ng PGE_2/mg creatinine, one can see a very significant increase of controls. I suggest that your patient has elevated urinary PGE_2 but did not collect his urine completely.

(1) J.Grill, J.C.Frölich, Bowden, R.E.et al., Am.J.Med.61: 43-51, 1976.

(2) Frölich J.C. et al., J. Clin.Invest. 55 : 763, 1975.

(3) Walker, L.A. et al.,Am.J.Physiol. 4 : F180, 1978.

J. Frölich With respect to our normal values of urinary PGE_2 in rats
I would like to refer you to our recent paper (Walker, L.A.
et al., Am.J.Physiol. <u>4</u> :F180, 1978). In this paper we have
shown that male Long Evans rats weighing between 200 and
250 g excrete 228 ± 53 ng (mean $\pm$ SE, n = 6). At that time
their urine osmolarity was 745 ± 55 mosm.
This additional parameter is of greatest importance for the
comparison of normal values, because our paper also shows
that changes in ADH-levels account for 80 % of the difference in urinary PGE_2 between normal rats and rats with
central diabetes insipidus. This latter group excretes 39 ± 5 ng/
24 hours only. ADH thus emerges as the single most important
requlator of urinary PGE_2-excretion.

J. Frölich The problem of separation of isotopes by HPLC was first
reported by me in 1976 (J.Frölich: Gaschromatography-mass
spectrometry of prostaglandins in "The Prostaglandins", Vol.3,
P.W. Ramwell, ed., Plenum Press, New York 1976, pp 1-39).
This problem not only applies to the separation of tritiated
and deuterated prostaglandins but also to the separation of
deuterated and labeled prostaglandins and thus can lead to
erroneously low or high values.

P. Lijnen Concerning the interpretation of the levels of urinary PGE_2
or $PGF_{2\alpha}$ excretions in healthy male and female subjects,
I would like to comment that these values have to be corrected
e.g. for sodium intake.
Indeed in 39 apparently normal subjects we found significant
(P < 0.001) lower values for $U_{PGE_2}V$ and $U_{PGF_{2\alpha}}.V$ in female
subjects compared to age-matched male subjects.

Using simple regression analysis we found a significant (P 0.05 positive correlation between $U_{PGE_2} \cdot V$ and $U_{PGF_{2\alpha}} \cdot V$ on the one side and on the other side the urinary sodium excretion ($U_{Na} \cdot V$) (r-value = 0.34; $P < 0.05$) and urinary potassium excretion ($U_K \cdot V$) (r = 0.38; $P < 0.05$).

Using multiple regression analysis $U_{PGE_2} \cdot V$ and $U_{PGF_{2\alpha}} \cdot V$ were significantly and independently related to $U_{Na} \cdot V$, $U_K \cdot V$ and sex. These results suggest, like other reports in the literature, that the renal primary prostaglandins E_2 and $F_{2\alpha}$ possess natriuretic actions and can have an important role in regulating sodium metabolism.

7 GC / MS MEASUREMENT OF 6-OXO-PGF$_{1\alpha}$ IN BIOLOGICAL FLUIDS

M. Claeys*, C. Van Hove, A. Duchateau and A.G. Herman

ABSTRACT

A selected ion monitoring method for the determination of 6-oxo PGF$_{1\alpha}$ in biological fluids has been worked out. In this method, biosynthetically pre-pared ^{2}H$_{7}$-6-oxo PGF$_{1\alpha}$ is used as internal standard. The method involves extraction, TLC purification and derivatization into the methyl ester, methoxime, trimethylsilyl ether derivatives by carrying out the methoximation first. Quantitative GC/MS analysis is performed in the electron impact mode by monitoring the $[M^{+\cdot} -(TMSOH + CH_3O^{\cdot})]$ – fragment ions.

The use of this method in the measurement of 6-oxo PGF$_{1\alpha}$ in serous fluids and in incubation media of serous tissues is described.

INTRODUCTION

During the past two years our laboratory has been concerned with the quanti-tative analysis of 6-oxo PGF$_{1\alpha}$, the stable end-product of prostacyclin(PGI$_2$), in body fluids. Reliable methodology for 6-oxo PGF$_{1\alpha}$ is needed in order to study the role of PGI$_2$ in endotoxin shock and to evaluate the in vivo effects of pharmacological agents on its biosynthesis, such as the effects of anti-oxydantia.

A radioimmunological method, developed by Salmon (1), has been selected for routine purposes and has recently been applied to measurements in total blood samples of endotoxin treated animals (2). Being aware of the dis-crepancies, often reported between radioimmunoassays (RIA) and chemical measurements (3), a reference method using isotope dilution (ID) and mass spectrometry (MS), i.e. selected ion monitoring (SIM) has been worked out in order to support RIA data. The technique of ID-MS may serve as a reference method as it can provide a specific and accurate means for determina-tion in biological fluids. The accuracy of ID-MS is based on the high specifi-

---

* Research associate of the Belgian "Nationaal Fonds voor Wetenschappelijk Onderzoek".

city of MS and on the exact control of recovery employing the principle of ID.
The present report describes our efforts on the development of an assay procedure for 6-oxo $PGF_{1\alpha}$.

MATERIALS AND METHODS

Materials

Chemicals and solvents were of analytical grade and were used without further
purification. The reference standard, 6-oxo $PGF_{1\alpha}$, was provided by
Dr. J.E. Pike of the Upjohn Company (Kalamazoo, Mi., U.S.A.).
$[5,6,8,9,11,12,14,15-^2H_8]$ - Arachidonic acid $(^2H_8-AA)$ was a gift from
Dr. D.H. Nugteren of Unilever Research (Vlaardingen, The Netherlands).

GC/MS Instrumentation and Analysis

A Finnigan 4000 gas chromatograph – mass spectrometer, interfaced with an
Incos 2000 data system, has been used in this study. GC was performed on
1.5 m x 2 mm i.d. glass column, containing 1 % Dexsil 300 on Gaschrom
Q100/120 mesh with a helium flow of 25 ml min^{-1} and using the jet separator
as GC/MS interface. Temperatures were : injector, 250°C; column, 240°C
and GC/MS interface, 230°C. The chemical ionization (CI) reagent gas,
methane, was added as make-up gas until the source pressure reached 40 Pa
(or 0.3 Torr). The MS conditions were : electron energy, 70eV; emission
current, 0.2 mA; ion source temperature, 230°C for electron impact (EI) and
180°C for CI. SIM was performed using a 4-channel programmable multiple
ion monitor (Promim) or using the Incos 2000 software. Quantitative SIM
analyses were performed in the EI mode at m/z 378 and 508, respectively
corresponding with the $[M^{+\cdot}-(2 \times TMSOH + C_5H_{11}\cdot)]$ - and $[M^{+\cdot}-(TMSOH + CH_3O\cdot)]$ - fragment ions (4) for monitoring 6-oxo $PGF_{1\alpha}$ and at 383 and
514 for monitoring its $^2H_7$- labeled analog.

Preparation of $^2H_7$-6-oxo $PGF_{1\alpha}$

$[5,6,8,9,11,12,14,15-^2H_8]$ prostaglandin endoperoxide $H_2 (^2H_8-PGH_2)$
was prepared by incubation of 2 mg $^2H_8-$ AA, mixed with a small amount of
$^{14}C-AA$ (800 000 dpm), with microsomes of ram seminal vesicles, following
the procedures described by Nugteren and Hazelhof (5); yield : 360 μg (18 %).
In a following step $[5,8,9,11,12,14,15-^2H_7]$ -6-oxo $PGF_{1\alpha} (^2H_7-6-oxo$

$PGF_{1\alpha}$) was obtained by incubation of the $^2H_8$-PGH_2 with pig aorta micro-somes using 0.4 mg protein μg^{-1} substrate and following the method by Johnson et al. (6); yield : 86.4 μg (24 %). The $^2H_7$-6-oxo $PGF_{1\alpha}$ was stored in ethanol at −20°C at a concentration of 10 $\mu g\ ml^{-1}$.

Quantitative Analysis

Standard curves were obtained with aqueous standard solutions, each containing known amounts of 6-oxo $PGF_{1\alpha}$, and by carrying these standards through the extraction, purification and derivatization steps. Quantitative calculations were based on peak height or on peak area ratios of the $[M^{+\cdot}-(TMSOH + CH_3O^\cdot)]$ – ion records of the compound of interest versus this of its $^2H_7$-labeled analog. Ratios for the standard mixtures were plotted against the concentra-tions in ng ml^{-1}, and an unweighted least squares linear regression analysis was performed. Using the regression parameters of the calibration curve, the unknown 6-oxo $PGF_{1\alpha}$ concentrations and their associated standard errors were estimated.

Extraction and purification procedure

After addition of the $^2H_7$-6-oxo $PGF_{1\alpha}$ (20 μl) containing approximately 200 ng, 1 volume of NaCl solution (0.9 %) and 2 volumes of ethanol, 2 ml of biological fluid was extracted with 5 ml of petroleum ether. The organic layer was discarded and after acidification with 2.3M citric acid (pH<3), the aqueous layer was extracted twice with 5 ml of chloroform. The combined extracts were evaporated to dryness under a nitrogen stream, the extraction residue was redissolved into a small volume of methanol: chloroform (1:1) and applied onto a precoated silicagel F (Merck) TLC plate. TLC analysis was performed using the double development technique, described by Sun et al. (7), with the organic phase of ethyl acetate : 2,2,4-trimethylpentane : acetic acid : water (110: 50: 20: 100) in a non-equilibrated tank. In order to localize 6-oxo $PGF_{1\alpha}$, 4 μg of authentic 6-oxo $PGF_{1\alpha}$ was applied separately on the TLC plate and was visualized after development by spraying with a 10 % ethanolic solution of phosphomolybdic acid and heating to 110°C. The corresponding 6-oxo $PGF_{1\alpha}$ zones, obtained from the biological extracts, were scraped off and eluted twice with 2 ml of methanol. The combined eluates were evaporated under nitrogen, the residue was redissolved into 0.5 ml of acidified water (0.03 M citric acid) and extracted twice with 1 ml of ether. The ether extracts were combined, dried under a nitrogen stream and subjected to derivatization.

Derivatization

Methyl ester formation. An ether solution of diazomethane (CH_2N_2) was prepared according to Fales et al. (8). For esterification, 0.5 ml of this solution was added to the residue, obtained after extraction or methoximation. The mixture was allowed to react for 5 min at room t° and evaporated to dryness.

Methoximation. Methoximation was carried out by reacting the residue, obtained after extraction or esterification, with 50 µl of a pyridine solution of methoxyamine – HCl salt (1mg ml^{-1}) for 1h30 min at 80°C. After completion of the methoximation, the reaction mixture was dried under nitrogen.

Trimethylsilylation. Trimethylsilylation was performed using 30 µl of N,O-bis (trimethylsilyl) trifluoroacetamide (BSTFA) and 10 µl of pyridine. The mixture was reacted for 30 min at 80°C and was evaporated to dryness. The derivatization residue was redissolved into 10 µl of hexane and aliquots of 2 µl were used for GC/MS analysis.

Biological samples

Rabbits of either sex (2 – 3 kg) were killed by a blow on the head and exsanguinated. Pericardial, pleural and peritoneal fluid was collected from the cavities and centrifuged at low speed (300 g) in order to remove the cells (9). Pieces of pericardium and peritoneum were removed, trimmed free of fat and put in ice cold Tris–HCl buffer (50 mM, pH 8). Tissues were incubated in 2 ml Tris–HCl buffer for 20 min at 37°C and removed from the incubation media before extraction was carried out.

RESULTS AND DISCUSSION

The GC/MS method applied for the measurement of 6-oxo $PGF_{1\alpha}$ includes the following sequential steps :

- isolation of the compound from the biological matrix by solvent extraction;
- purification and fractionation by TLC;
- derivative formation in order to enhance volatility;
- GC/MS analysis.

It is obvious that each of these steps has to be optimized if nanogram quantities need to be determined.

Isolation of 6-oxo PGF$_{1\alpha}$

For the extraction of 6-oxo PGF$_{1\alpha}$ we used non-precipitating amounts of ethanol (50 % v/v), following the procedure described by Unger et al.(10). These authors showed that poor recoveries found in the extraction of prostaglandins from blood result from binding of the prostaglandin onto precipitated serum albumin. Since 6-oxo PGF$_{1\alpha}$ is one of the more polar prostaglandins, protein precipitation was avoided.

Purification by TLC

The extract containing 6-oxo PGF$_{1\alpha}$ requires purification before derivatization and GC/MS measurement can be carried out. Preliminary attempts to analyze crude extracts by GC/MS after derivatization were unsuccesful. The crude prostaglandin extract was purified and fractionated by TLC on silicagel F, using the organic phase of ethyl acetate – 2,2,4-trimethylpentane-acetic acid – water (110: 50: 20: 100) in a non-equilibrated tank and applying the double development technique as described by Sun et al.(7). Under the conditions used, 6-oxo PGF$_{1\alpha}$ elutes as a sharp zone and is well resolved from PGF$_{2\alpha}$, PGE$_2$ and from a red coloured haem zone, which was always present in our crude biological extracts and co-chromatographed with PGF$_{2\alpha}$ thereby facilitating the location of the 6-oxo PGF$_{1\alpha}$ zone on the TLC plates. In following steps, the 6-oxo PGF$_{1\alpha}$ zone was eluted from the silicagel with methanol and the extract was partitioned in the system water (0.03 M citric acid)-ether in order to remove the minute amounts of silicagel, which were carried over with methanol elution. Attempts to analyze the methanol extract directly by GC/MS after derivatization failed, probably because silicagel interfered in the derivative formation. The recovery of the analytical procedure, including extraction, TLC purification and partition was determined using ^{3}H$_7$-6-oxo PGF$_{1\alpha}$(4500 dpm) and a pool of serous fluid to which non-labeled 6-oxo PGF$_{1\alpha}$ was added to a concentration of 21.9 ng ml^{-1}; it was estimated to be 36.7 % (SD = 1.0 %; N = 5).

Formation of the methyl ester, methoxime, TMS-ether derivative

The applicability of gas phase methods for the determination of sub-microgram quantities of prostaglandins depends to a large extent on the ready conversion into a volatile derivative. With regard to the derivatization of 6-oxo $PGF_{1\alpha}$ and structurally related compounds, containing both the 6-oxo and the 9-hydroxyl functions, difficulties have been reported by Sun and Taylor (11). Preliminary attempts to derivatize 6-oxo $PGF_{1\alpha}$ at the 100 ng level and following the conventional sequence of carrying out the methyl ester formation first, resulted in poor SIM responses on subsequent GC/MS analysis. In an attempt to optimize the yield of methyl ester, methoxime, TMS-ether derivative we reversed the sequence of the derivatization reactions by carrying out the methoximation first (Scheme 1). At the 100 ng level this proce-

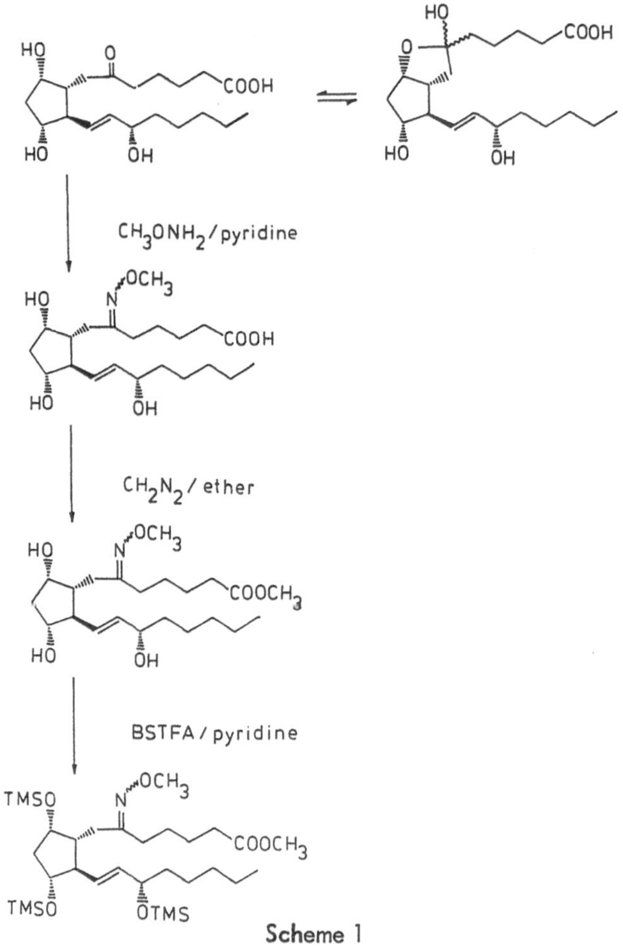

Scheme 1

dure resulted in a 5-fold increase in derivative yield. This result can be rationalized by the fact that 6-oxo $PGF_{1\alpha}$ can also be present in the lactol form, in which the hemi-ketal function may be trapped by methylation in the reaction with diazomethane, making the resulting ketal less accessible to methoximation in a following derivatization step.

GC/MS analysis

Selection of the ionization method. Two available ionization methods, i.e. EI and CI using methane as reagent gas, were compared for sensitive MS analysis. The EI and CI (methane) spectra of the 6-oxo $PGF_{1\alpha}$, methyl ester, methoxime TMS-ether derivative, as obtained under our experimental conditions, are given in figures 1 and 2. Extensive fragmentation can be noticed in the EI mode, mainly resulting in abundant ions in the lower mass region. In contrast, CI(methane) shows a more simple pattern, yielding no

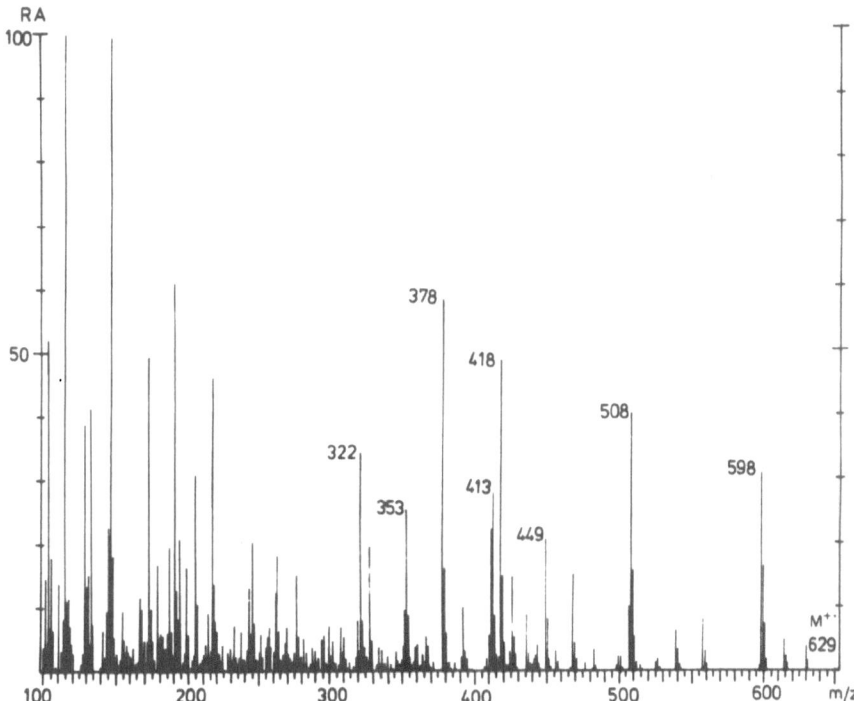

Fig. 1 : EI mass spectrum of 6-oxo $PGF_{1\alpha}$ methyl ester, methoxime, TMS-ether.

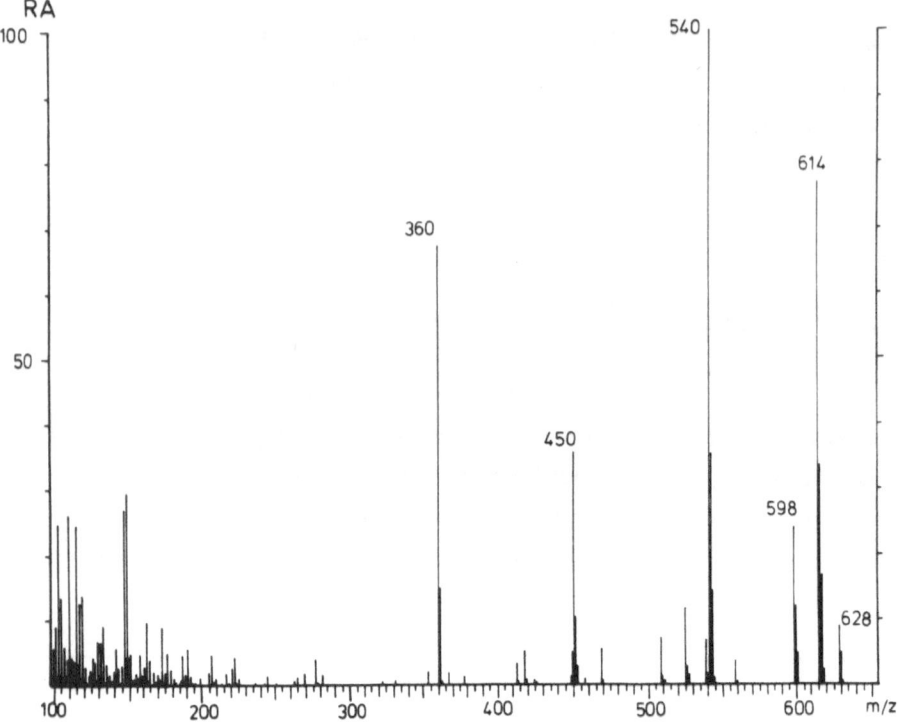

MH$^+$-ion(m/z 630), but a few relatively abundant ions at m/z 614,540,
450 and 360, respectively corresponding with the loss of methane and with
the consecutive loss of 1,2 and 3 trimethylsilanol(TMSOH) molecules.
Using SIM, the CI(methane) mode however, did not appear to be suitable
for detecting low quantities in the nanogram range, probably because the
ionization efficiency in this mode is low. It should be stressed that relative
ion abundance in a mass spectrum, is not the determining factor for sensitivity of SIM in that particular ionization mode. The important criteria are
the absolute ion currents, which can be compared by measuring a fixed
amount of the compound of interest in the different modes of ionization.
In the comparison carried out by single ion monitoring and for which the
most abundant ion above m/z 300 was selected (m/z 378 for EI and m/z 540
for CI(methane), 1 ng of authentic 6-oxo PGF$_{1\alpha}$ derivative could be detected with a S/N of 5/1 in the EI mode, whereas in the CI(methane) mode,

an amount of 10 ng was still undetectable. As a result, EI was employed in subsequent SIM analyses. In order to ensure the specificity of the detection, a second ion in the higher mass region was monitored at m/z 508. Using the m/z 508 trace and a sample size of 2 ml, the limit of detection was 5 ng ml^{-1}. This concentration could be detected with a S/N of 5/1, yielded a signal which was about twice the size of the blank or the contribution due to $^2H_0$-form present in the internal standard and could be determined with a standard error of 1.2 ng ml^{-1}.

Preparation of $^2H_7$-6-oxo PGF$_{1\alpha}$. The internal standard, $^2H_7$-6-oxo PGF$_{1\alpha}$ was prepared from $^2H_8$-AA by a 2 step biochemical procedure: in a first step, $^2H_8$-AA was converted into $^2H_8$-PGH$_2$ using microsomes of ram seminal vesicles (5), which in a second step was transformed into $^2H_7$-6-oxo PGF$_{1\alpha}$ using pig aorta microsomes (6). The $^2H_7$-6-oxo PGF$_{1\alpha}$ thus obtained, contained 4.6 % of the natural $^2H_0$-form. The occurrence of this non-deuterated 6-oxo PGF$_{1\alpha}$ should originate from dilution with $^2H_0$-AA, which was present in the free form in our non-washed microsome preparations or was released by them during incubation.

Since $^2H_7$-6-oxo PGF$_{1\alpha}$ contains a deuterium label at the enolizable 5-position, exchange of this labile deuterium atom could occur during the sample work-up. Experiments revealed that loss of label does not occur during the extraction and purification procedures. SIM analyses, in which the ions corresponding with $M^{+\cdot}$-(TMSOH + CH$_3$O$^\cdot$) were monitored, were performed on 200 ng of $^2H_7$-6-oxo PGF$_{1\alpha}$, carried through the extraction and purification steps, as well as on the same amount of $^2H_7$-6-oxo PGF$_{1\alpha}$, which was directly derivatized. The analyses showed a similar isotopic pattern for the two types of samples (fig.3). The analyses also demonstrated that the m/z 508 ion is shifted to m/z 514 and to some extent also to m/z 513, which probably corresponds with $M^{+\cdot}$-(TMSO$^2H_0$ + CH$_3$O$^\cdot$). This shift of 6 amu indicates that the biosynthetically prepared $^2H_7$-6-oxo PGF$_{1\alpha}$ only contains 6 deuterium atoms and has already lost a labile deuterium atom during its preparation. The EI mass spectrum of the $^2H_7$-6-oxo PGF$_{1\alpha}$ derivative (not shown) further confirms this conclusion; the highest mass ion is at m/z 614, which is due to the loss of a CH$_3$O$^\cdot$-moiety and which again corresponds with a shift of 6 amu. Loss of label from biosynthetically prepared deuterium-labeled prostaglandins has been described for PGD$_2$, where loss of deuterium occurs at the 12-position(12, 13).

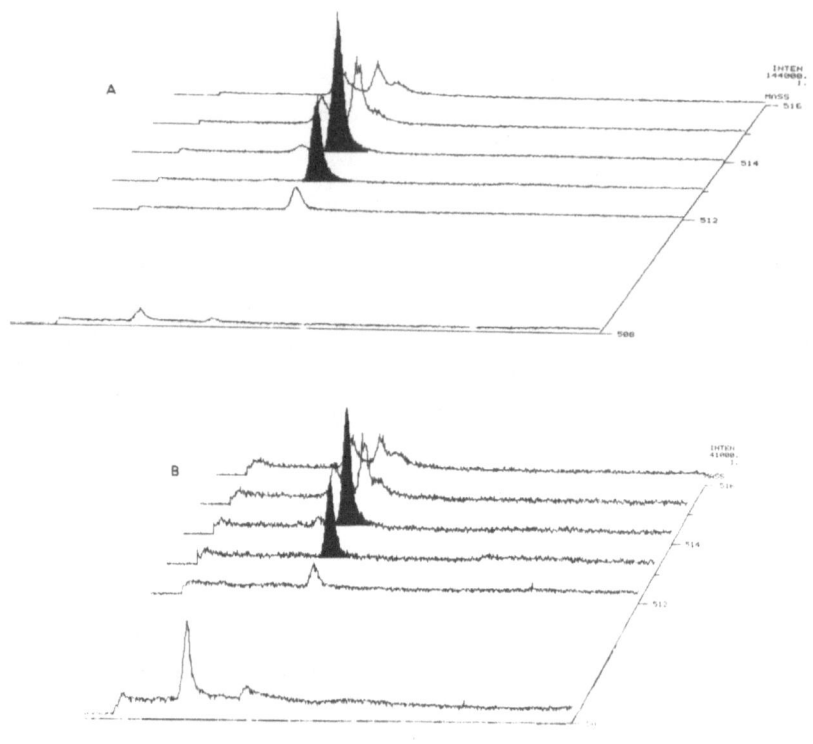

Fig.3 : SIM analyses obtained on 200 ng of $^2H_7$-6-oxo $PGF_{1\alpha}$ directly
derivatized (A) and on the same amount of internal standard carried
through the extraction and purification steps (B).

Problems have also been reported for $^2H_5$-6-oxo $PGF_{1\alpha}$ methyl ester, used
by Pace Asciak and prepared by a combination of enzymic and chemical
techniques (14,15). This material resulted in poor precision, which was
ascribed to the possibly unpredictable ratio between the $[M^{+\cdot}-(TMSOH + CH_3O^\cdot)]$ - and $[M^{+\cdot}-(TMSO^2H_0 + CH_3O^\cdot)]$ - fragment ions. In our
preparation however, the ratio $[M^{+\cdot}-(TMSOH + CH_3O^\cdot)] / [M^{+\cdot}-(TMSO^2H_0 + CH_3O^\cdot)]$ remained stable when multiple analyses were performed on the same sample, indicating that the material can safely be used
as internal standard ([m/z 514] / [m/z 513] = 7.6; SD=1.6; N= 5).

<u>Quantitative analysis</u>. A series of 5 aqueous standards, covering the con-
centration range of interest (10–100 ng ml^{-1}), was used to construct a calibration curve. A typical curve is shown in fig.4 in order to demonstrate the
linearity and the precision. The curves were obtained by unweighted least
squares linear regression based on previous research, which indicated that
this type of statistical analysis can be employed with stable isotope labeled
internal standards and for a 10–fold range of x–values because the errors
associated with the y–values are approximately constant (16). Using the
regression line(fig.4) in reverse, a standard error of 1.2 ng ml^{-1} could be

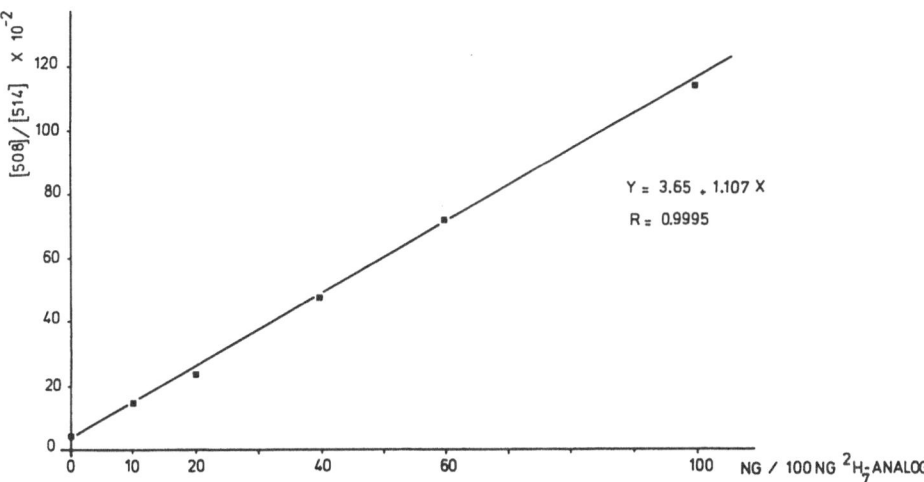

Fig.4 : Calibration curve prepared from five 2 ml aqueous standards containing approximately 200 ng $^2H_7$–analog

estimated, corresponding quite well with the variation observed when multiple
samples of a pool of peritoneal fluid were analyzed(concentration: 28.0 ng ml^{-1};
SD=1.3 ng ml^{-1}; N = 4). For quantitative analysis, the $[m/z\ 508]$ /
$[m/z\ 514]$ ratio was used. Despite the fact that the ion at m/z 378 allows
a more sensitive detection, it could not be employed for precise quantitation because significant interference occurred on the m/z 383–trace, used
for monitoring the internal standard. It is also obvious that it is not
feasible to construct a new calibration curve in each series of experiments
by subjecting a number of aqueous standards to the entire time–consuming

work-up procedures. When an old calibration was used however, its validity was checked by re-analyzing 1 or 2 aqueous standards.

Applications

In a previous study from our laboratory, we demonstrated that the serous membranes (pericardium, peritoneum and pleura) of the rabbit have a significant capacity to biosynthetize PGI_2 (17). A typical radiochromatogram, obtained on peritoneum which was incubated in Tris-HCl buffer in the presence of ^{14}C-AA, is given in fig.5, in order to show the 2 main transformation products of AA: 6-oxo $PGF_{1\alpha}$, the stable end-product of PGI_2 and a compound, which co-chromatographs with 12-L-hydroxy-5,8,10,14-eicosatetraenoic acid (12-HETE).

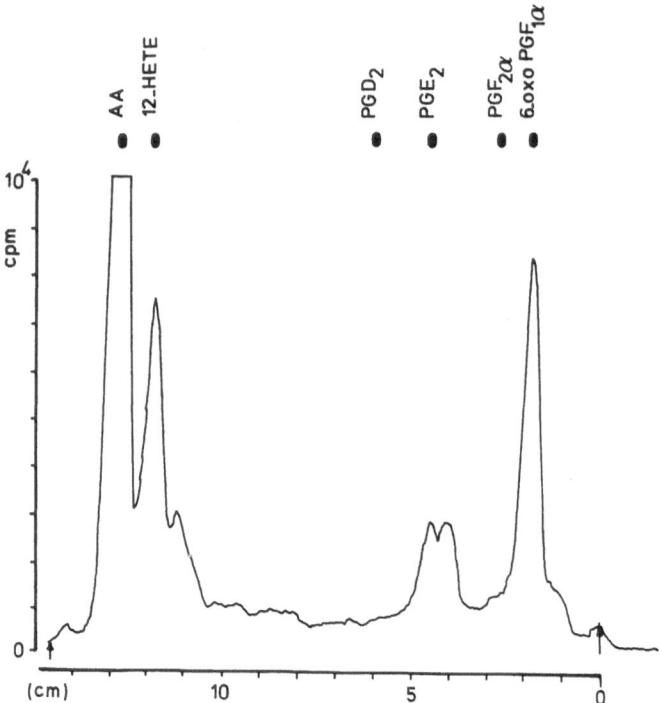

Fig.5 : Radiochromatogram, obtained on peritoneum (213 mg), which was incubated in 2 ml of Tris-HCl buffer (50 mM, pH8) containing ^{14}C-AA (5.4 µg, 1 µCi).

The present assay was applied to the analysis of media in which tissues had been incubated without addition of exogenous AA, and to the analysis of serous fluids. The 6-oxo $PGF_{1\alpha}$ levels found are given in table 1 and a typical analysis, obtained on peritoneal fluid, is shown in fig.6. The results in table 1 demonstrate that the serous tissues can generate significant

Table 1   6-oxo $PGF_{1\alpha}$ levels in serous fluids and in incubation media of serous tissues of rabbits[a].

Animal	Biological fluid	level(ng ml^{-1})
Rabbit 1	pericardial fluid	12.9
	peritoneal fluid	22.7
	pleural fluid	10.9
	pericardium incubate	30.6
	peritoneum incubate	56.4
Rabbit 2	peritoneal fluid	27.9
Rabbit 3	peritoneal fluid	18.7

[a]The biological fluids were assayed in duplicate and each of the duplicate samples was injected into the GC/MS two or three times. The values from these multiple injections were then averaged to obtain a value for a specimen. The values for duplicate samples were averaged to obtain a final value for the biological fluid.

amounts of 6-oxo $PGF_{1\alpha}$; peritoneal tissue has about twice the activity of pericardial tissue, which is consistent with results from biosynthesis experiments with exogenous ^{14}C-AA (17). The high concentrations of 6-oxo $PGF_{1\alpha}$ found in the serous fluids indicate that PGI_2 has been released. A source for the high levels of 6-oxo $PGF_{1\alpha}$ in fluid collected from the serous cavities are most likely the serous tissues. Whether these membranes also generate PGI_2 in vivo however, and contribute to circulating PGI_2, as shown for the lung (18,19), remains to be established.

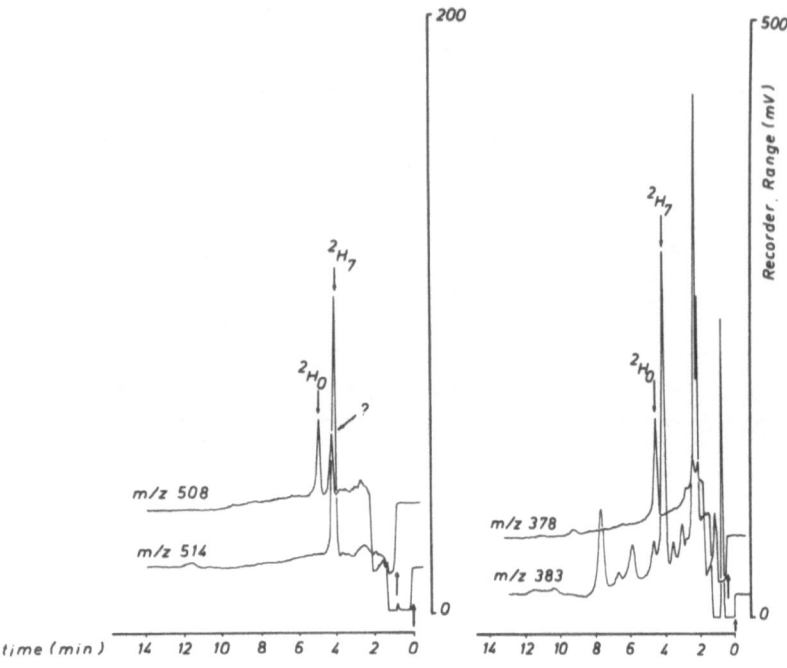

Fig.6 : Typical SIM analysis, obtained on peritoneal fluid of a rabbit.

Conclusions

Our GC/MS method as it stands now allows determination of 6-oxo PGF$_{1\alpha}$ in the nanogram range with acceptable precision. The demonstrated sensitivity was adequate for measuring 6-oxo PGF$_{1\alpha}$ levels in serous fluids and in incubation media of serous tissues. Increased sensitivity however will be needed for quantitation in blood, where subnanogram amounts have been demonstrated (19).

ACKNOWLEDGEMENTS

This work was supported by the Belgian National Medical Research Foundation (FGWO) through grant 3.9001.79 and by the Belgian Government through grant 77/81-1110.

REFERENCES

1. SALMON JA : A radioimmunoassay for 6–keto–prostaglandin $F_{1\alpha}$. Prostaglandins 15 : 383 – 397, 1978.

2. BULT H, BEETENS J, VERCRUYSSE P, HERMAN AG : Blood levels of 6–keto–$PGF_{1\alpha}$, the stable metabolite of prostacyclin during endotoxin–induced hypotension. Arch.Int. Pharmacodyn. 236: 285–286, 1978.

3. GRANSTROM E : Radioimmunoassay of prostaglandins. Prostaglandins 15 : 3 – 17, 1978.

4. COCKERILL AF, MALLEN DNB, OSBORNE DJ, BOOT JR, DAWSON W : Mass spectral characterization of 6–oxo $PGF_{1\alpha}$. Biomed. Mass Spectrom. 4: 358 – 363, 1977.

5. NUGTEREN DH, HAZELHOF E : Isolation and properties of intermediates in prostaglandin biosynthesis. Biochim. Biophys. Acta 326: 448 – 461, 1973.

6. JOHNSON RA, MORTON DR, KINNER JH, GORMAN RR, McGUIRE JC, SUN FF, WHITTAKER N, BUNTING S, SALMON JA, MONCADA S, VANE JR : The chemical structure of prostaglandin X (prostacyclin). Prostaglandins 12: 915 – 928, 1976.

7. SUN FF., CHAPMAN JP., McGUIRE JC: Metabolism of prostaglandin endoperoxide in animal tissues. Prostaglandins 14 : 1055 – 1074, 1977.

8. FALES HM, JAOUNI TM, BABASHAK JF : Simple device for preparing ethereal diazomethane without resorting to codestillation. Anal.Chem. 45 : 2302 – 2303, 1973.

9. VELO GP, DUNN CJ, GIROUD JP, TIMSIT J, WILLOUGHBY DA : The distribution of prostaglandins in inflammatory exudate. J.Pathol. 111 : 149 – 158, 1973.

10. UNGER WG, STAMFORD IF, BENNETT A : Extraction of prostaglandins from human blood. Nature 233 : 336 – 337, 1971.

11. SUN FF, TAYLOR BM : Metabolism of prostacyclin in rat. Biochem. 17: 4096 – 4101, 1978.

12. SAEED ABDEL-HALIM M, HAMBERG M, SJOQVIST B, ANGGARD E : Identification of prostaglandin D_2 as a major prostaglandin in homogenates of rat brain. Prostaglandins 14 : 633 – 643, 1977.

13. ROBERTS LJ II, LEWIS RA, OATES JO, AUSTEN KF : Prostaglandin, tromboxane, and 12-hydroxy-5,8,10,14-eicosatetraenoic acid production by ionophore - stimulated rat serosal mast cells. Biochim. Biophys. Acta 575 : 185 - 192, 1979.

14. PACE ASCIAK CR : Deuterium isotope dilution method for the specific measurement of 6-keto-prostaglandin $F_{1\alpha}$ by mass fragmentography. Anal. Biochem. 81 : 251 - 255, 1977

15. PACE ASCIAK CR : The 6 [9] oxy cyclase pathway of prostaglandin endoperoxide metabolism, in : Chemistry, biochemistry and pharmacological activity of prostanoids, Roberts SM, Scheinmann F (eds), Oxford, Pergamon Press, 1979, p.313 - 325.

16. CLAEYS M, MARKEY SP, MAENHAUT W : Variance analysis of error in selected ion monitoring assays using various internal standards. A practical study case, Biomed. Mass Spectrom. 4 : 122 - 128, 1977.

17. HERMAN AG, CLAEYS M, MONCADA S, VANE JR : Biosynthesis of prostacyclin (PGI_2) and 12L-hydroxy-5,8,10,14-eicosatetraenoic acid (HETE) by pericardium, pleura, peritoneum and aorta of the rabbit. Prostaglandins 18 : 439 - 453, 1979.

18. GRYGLEWSKI RJ, KORBUT R, OCETKIEWICZ AC : Generation of prostacyclin by lungs in vivo and its release into the arterial circulation. Nature 273 : 765 - 767, 1978.

19. HENSBY CN, DOLLERY CT, BARNES PJ, DARGIE H : Production of 6-oxo $PGF_{1\alpha}$ by human lung in vivo. The Lancet 1162 - 1163,1978.

DISCUSSION

J. Salmon   Have you used other gases for chemical ionization mass spectrometry, for example have you used ammonia?

M. Claeys   We have only evaluated methane as a reagent gas for chemical ionization, because for most organic molecules containing C, H and O, the ionization efficiency with methane is usually larger than with isobutane and ammonia. Other reasons for not using ammonia are that it is a very reactive gas, which corrodes the gas inlet system and shortens the filament life-time and which as such make it very in-convenient for routine measurements.

J. Salmon   What is the general concensus about how much deuterated internal standard should be added? Should it only act as an internal standard or should it act as a carrier as well? Do you need less deuterated standard when capillary columns are used?

M. Claeys   For quantitative GC/MS work we try to use an amount of labeled internal standard which is lower than the 10-fold of the amount of compound to be measured. Our reason for doing so is that, for a 10-fold range of (compound)/(internal standard) ratios, a calibration curve can be constructed by applying an unweighted least squares linear regression analysis because the errors associated with the mass spectral response ratios are approximately constant. One should also keep in mind that a higher amount of labeled internal standard may increase the detection limit. In our particular 6-oxo $PGF_{1\alpha}$ assay for example, we use 100 ng ml^{-1} of labeled analog, which contains about 5 % of the $^2H_0$-form and which corres-ponds with a blank of 5 ng ml^{-1}. Ideally, the deuterated standard should also act as a carrier in order to correct for the adsorptive losses, which are likely to occur in the low nanogram range.

With regard to your question concerning the amount of
standard necessary when capillary columns are used, I don't
see a difference with packed columns. The advantages of using
capillary columns instead of packed columns lie in their
inertness and in their better chromatographic resolution.

H.W.Seyberth   Do you have any experience with PGE_2 analysis using capillary columns?

M. Claeys   No, we haven't.

H.W. Seyberth   What kind of interface do you use?

M. Claeys   With our GC/MS system we have 3 possibilities for inter-
facing : for packed columns, we use a glass jet separator
in the case of electron impact ionization and a direct glass
line of 0.5 mm i.d. when chemical ionization is applied,
whereas for capillary columns, we use a glass coated metal
tube of 0.25 mm i.d.

B.B.Vargaftig   Have you tried to prevent release of arachidonic acid from
ram seminal vesicle and for aortic microsomes with phospholipase A_2 inhibitors ?

M. Claeys   No, we never considered it but it may be worth trying. I
should mention that there are methods described in the
literature by which low blank deuterated internal standards
can be prepared. In the procedures, the microsomes are
washed with acetone or with buffer containing bovine serum
albumin, which traps the free arachidonic acid.

E. Schell-   Passing from methodological to clinical considerations, have
Frederick   you been able to study human serous fluids ?

M. Claeys   No, we haven't.

8 METABOLITE MEASUREMENT AS AN INDEX OF PROSTAGLANDIN SYNTHESIS IN VIVO

A.R. Brash

1. INTRODUCTION

The analysis of metabolite levels is often the most appropriate method for the monitoring of prostaglandin biosynthesis in vivo. The factors which weigh against the measurement of the primary cyclo-oxygenase products are their de novo synthesis on the handling of any tissue, their extremely fast metabolism and in some cases their chemical instability. Bioassay methods can overcome these difficulties but there are many instances, especially in human studies, when one is limited to the collection of peripheral plasma samples or urine. Under these circumstances the levels of a biologically inactive metabolite can provide a good index of endogenous biosynthesis.

The metabolite measurements reported below were all performed with quantitative analysis by selected ion monitoring GC-MS. The analysis of low level samples by GC-MS presents many technical difficulties. Some of these arise during method development when an appropriate internal standard must be prepared; others relate to the stringent purifications often required prior to the GC-MS analysis itself. Most of the technical aspects of this paper deal with these two problem areas. The development and application of an assay for 5α, 7α-dihydroxy-11-ketotetranor-prostane 1,16, dioic acid is described. This compound is the major urinary metabolite of $PGF_{1\alpha}$ and $PGF_{2\alpha}$ in man, and is referred to below as PGF-M. The compound exists in a pH-dependent equilibrium between a diacid and corresponding δ-lactone form (Figure 1). Although the formation of the δ-lactone could complicate a quantitative analysis in fact it proved to be extremely useful in the selective purification of PGF-M from other urinary acids.

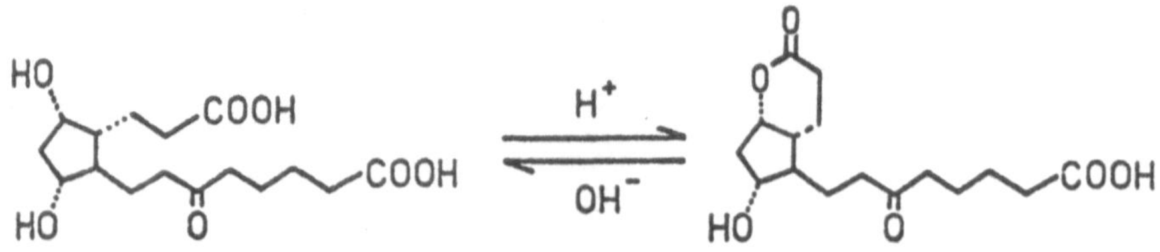

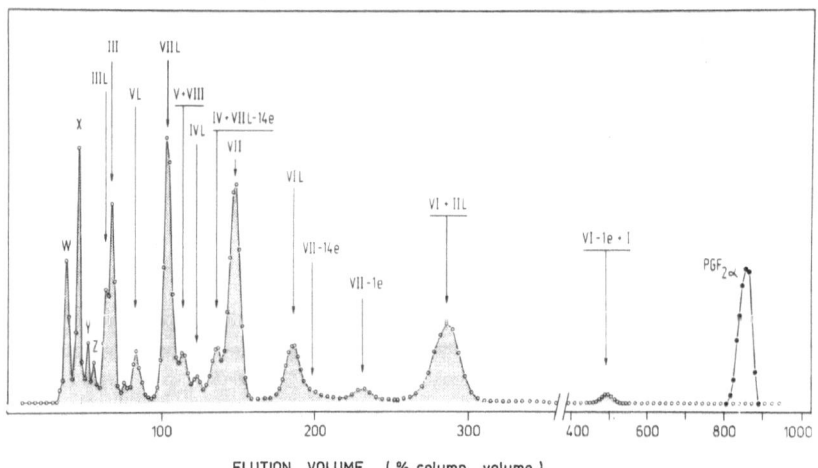

Figure 1. The dioic acid and corresponding δ-lactone forms of PGF-M.

2. DEVELOPMENT OF AN ASSAY FOR PGF-M

2.1 Preparation of [5β-^{3}H] PGF-M methyl ester

This compound was isolated from the urine of rats dosed with 10 mg of [5β-^{3}H] PGF$_{2\alpha}$ (1). Following extraction of the urine with Amberlite XAD-2 and treatment of the methanol eluate with diazomethane, the ra-diolabeled metabolites were separated by reversed phase liquid-gel chromatography (Figure 2) (2). Further purification was achieved using straight-phase liquid-gel chromatography for preparative scale separa-tions (1,3). Prior to analysis of GC-MS the metabolites were purified

Figure 2. Separation of the methyl esters of radiolabeled metabolites and unlabeled PGF$_{2\alpha}$ methyl ester (1 mg added to the urine extract). The structures of the metabolites are given in Figure 4. The letter L denotes a δ-lactone derivative and 1e denotes a C-1 ethyl ester.

Compounds W,X,Y,Z were identified as metabolites in the free acid form (present due to incomplete methylation of the extract). Column: Lipidex 1000 (44 X 2 cm). Solvent: water/methanol/butanol/chloroform, 60/40/7/3 (by volume).

by TLC of their t-butyldimethylsilyl (t-BDMS) ether derivatives. This method proved very effective for the separation of the metabolites, and in addition, it gave some clues to the structure of the compounds. This followed from the observation that the more t-BDMS groups were in the molecule, the higher the R_F value on TLC; the δ-lactone derivatives were found to have lower R_F values than the corresponding methyl ester derivatives. An example is shown in Figure 3, in which the compounds in the peak labeled V + VIII from Figure 1 (and the contaminating compounds from the shoulders of the adjacent peaks VII L and IV L) were converted to the t-BDMS ether derivatives and subjected to TLC. The metabolic pathways of $PGF_{2\alpha}$ were determined (Figure 4) (4). Radiochemically pure PGF-M methyl ester was isolated and used as a standard.

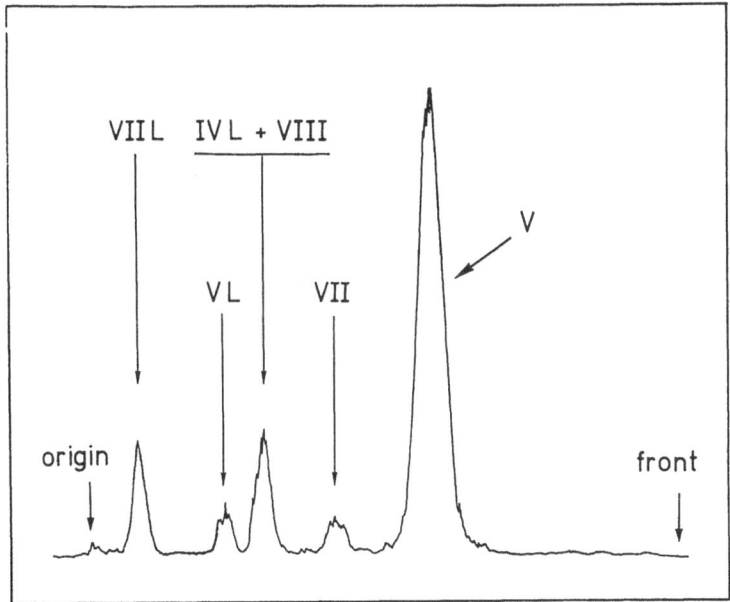

Figure 3. Thin layer radiochromatogram of the methyl ester t-BDMS ether derivatives of the compounds in peak V + VIII (Figure 2). The structures of the metabolites are given in Figure 4. The letter L denotes a δ-lactone derivative. Silica gel 60, solvent system, heptane/ethyl acetate 60:40, v/v.

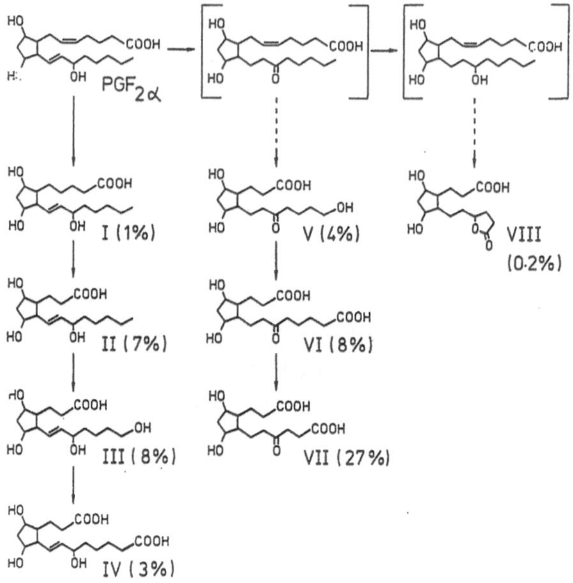

126

Figure 4. Urinary metabolites of PGF$_{2\alpha}$ in the male Wistar rat. The percentage of the administered radioactivity accounted for by each metabolite is given in parentheses.

2.2 Preparation of [5β-^{3}H,4,6,6-^{2}H$_3$] PGF-M methyl ester

The starting material was unlabeled PGE$_2$. The first reaction involved alkali-catalyzed deuteration of C-8 and C-10 in the PGE$_2$ molecule (1) using a reaction which was originally described as a means of preparation of 8-iso-PGE$_2$ (5). At equilibrium the mixture of PGE$_2$ and 8-iso-PGE$_2$ is about 9:1 in favor of the naturally occurring isomer. Following sodium borohydride reduction of the reaction mixture, four PGF isomers were obtained. The deuterium atoms at C-8 and C-10 are now in chemically non-exchangeable and metabolically stable positions. Deuterated PGF$_{2\alpha}$ was isolated by reversed-phase liquid-gel chromatography. This material was mixed with [9β-^{3}H] PGF$_{2\alpha}$ and administered to a Rhesus monkey. The required deuterated metabolite was isolated from the urine by liquid-gel chromatography.

In the reaction scheme above, the sodium borohydride reduction step affords the opportunity for the introduction of a tritium atom or a fourth deuterium at C-9. The resulting $[^2H, ^3H]$ PGF$_{2\alpha}$ can be converted in vivo or in vitro to any PGF metabolite and used as internal standard in a quantitative GC-MS analysis. The corresponding PGE or PGD compounds should also be amenable to analysis (after borohydride reduction) with this type of internal standard (Figure 5). Chemical transformation of PGF$_{2\alpha}$ to thromboxane B$_2$ (6) and prostacyclin (7) has been described. Use of these reactions opens the route to the preparation of any $[^2H, ^3H]$ TxB$_2$ or $[^2H, ^3H]$ PGI$_2$ metabolite (Figure 5). Dr. Pierre Falardeau and myself have used this method for the preparation of milligram quantities of $[^2H, ^3H]$ 6-keto-PGF$_{1\alpha}$. Using this approach it is possible to prepare any desired metabolite in sufficient yield for use in a GC-MS assay.

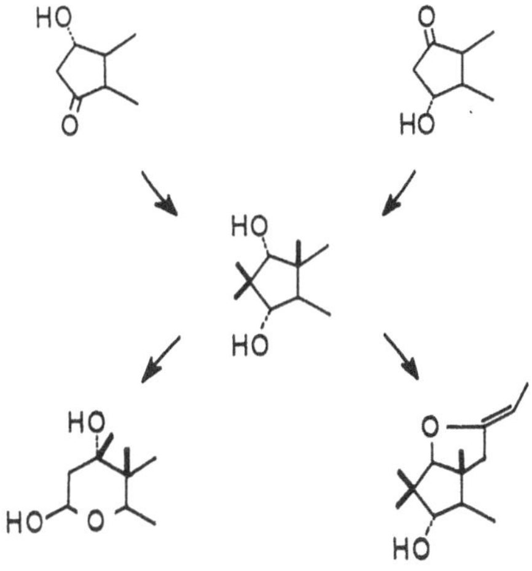

Figure 5. Applications of $[8,10,10-^2H_3]$ PGF$_{2\alpha}$ in prostaglandin analyses (see text). During the preparation of the PGF$_{2\alpha}$ from PGE$_2$ it can be labeled with a fourth deuterium or a tritium atom at C-9 (illustrated in the Figure for TxB$_2$).

2.3 Properties of PGF-M used in a purification method

2.3.1 Alkaline hydrolysis of the methyl ester

Treatment of the methyl ester (i.e. the 1,16-dimethyl ester) with pH 10 buffer caused selective hydrolysis of the C-1 ester group. Treatment

128

with 0.5N NaOH gave the diacid derivative (Figure 6). When the pH 10 hydrolysis product was esterified with ethyl iodide, subsequent mass spectrometric analysis proved that exclusively the 1-ethyl ester, 16-methyl ester derivative was formed (1). The reaction is shown in Figure 7.

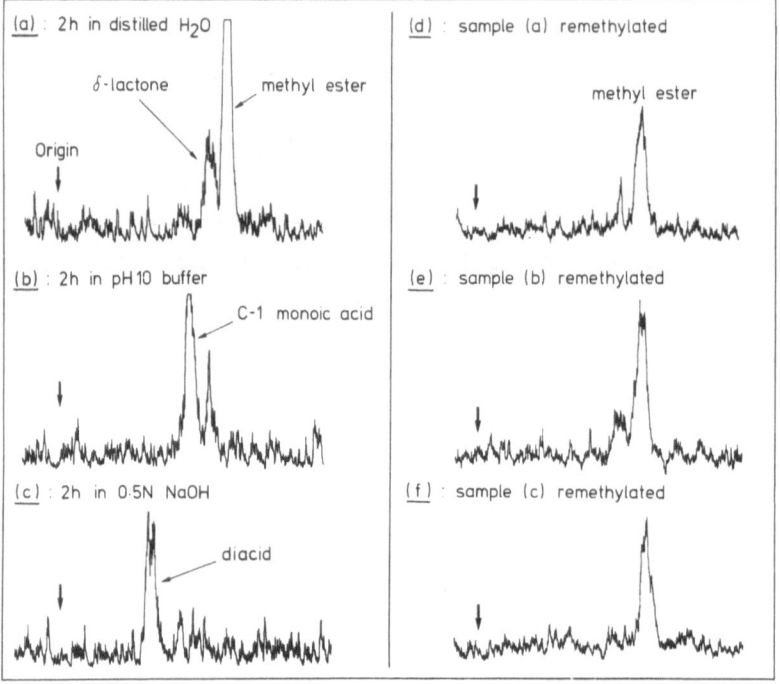

Figure 6. Thin layer radiochromatograms of the products obtained by hydrolysis and remethylation of PGF-M methyl ester. TLC solvent system: organic layer of ethyl acetate/methanol/water/acetic acid, 110/40/100/5 (by volume).

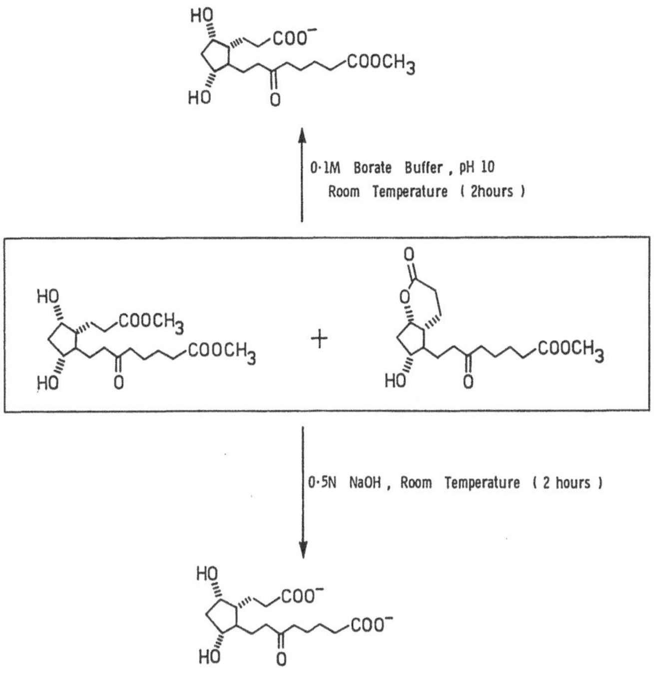

Figure 7. Alkaline hydrolysis of PGF-M and its δ-lactone derivative.

2.3.2 Rate of formation of the δ-lactone

When aliquots of the pH 10 hydrolysis product were added to acidic buffer solutions, a time-dependent and pH-dependent change in extraction into dichloroethane was observed. This change in partition coefficient is due to the formation of the δ-lactone derivative from the 5-hydroxy acid at acidic pH. As shown in Figure 8, lactonization was complete after 5 minutes at pH 1 or 1 hour at pH 2 whereas there was no reaction at pH 5 over the course of 2 hours.

2.3.3 Rate of hydrolysis of the δ-lactone

It was found that the δ-lactone was fairly stable at pH 8 whereas it was completely hydrolyzed to the "open-chain" acid after 2 hours at pH 10 (Figure 9).

130

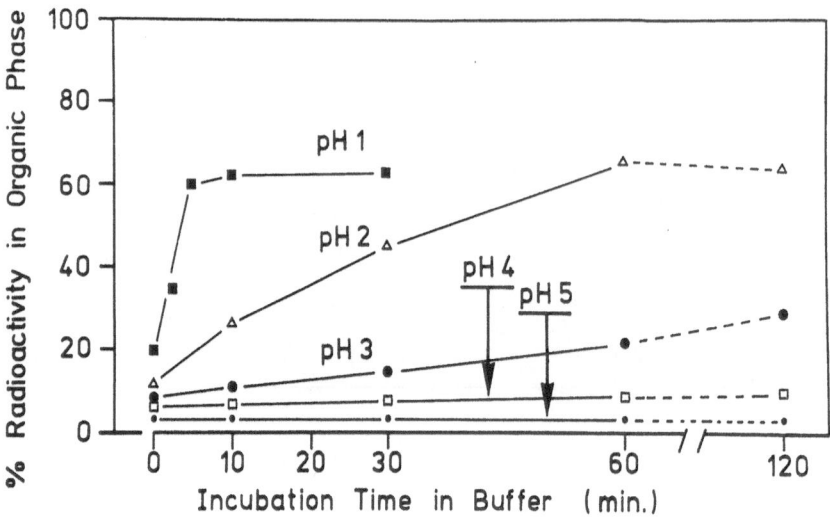

Figure 8. Rate of formation of the δ-lactone derivate of PGF-M as a function of pH and time. (The sample of C-1 acid, C-16 methyl ester used in this experiment probably contained some PGF-M diacid derivative. Hence the extraction was only 65% after lactonization compared with 90% found for pure δ-lactone C-16 methyl ester in Figure 9).

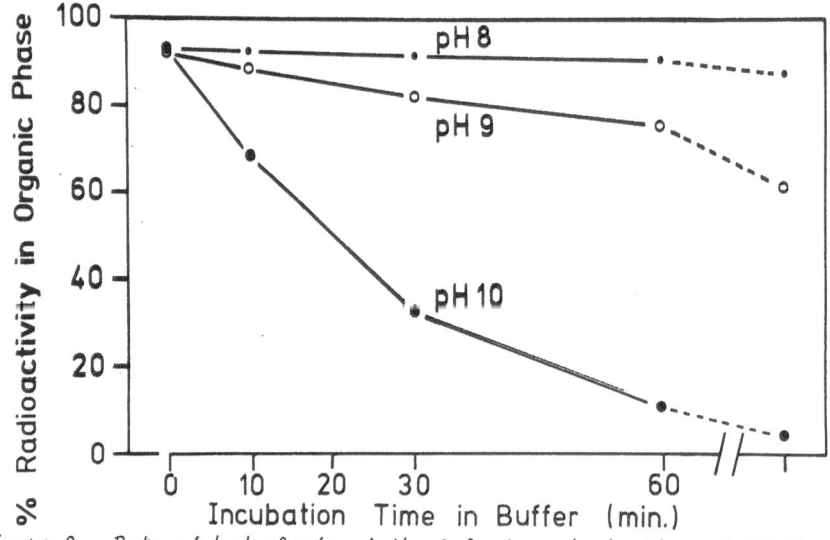

Figure 9. Rate of hydrolysis of the δ-lactone derivative of PGF-M as a function of pH and time.

2.3.4 *Quantitative conversion of the δ-lactone to the methyl ester*

Treatment of the δ-lactone derivative with diazomethane was found to give variable yields of the corresponding methyl ester. An alternative esterification procedure would be the use of tetramethylammonium hydroxide/methyl iodide (8). Since this reaction includes the presence of a base, initial treatment of the δ-lactone with tetramethylammonium hydroxide in methanol can be used to open the δ-lactone ring and allow quantitative esterification upon addition of the aprotic solvent dimethylacetamide and methyl iodide. The results of such an experiment as shown in Figure 10. The products were converted to their t-BDMS ether derivatives prior to analysis by TLC; t-BDMS formation was found to be necessary in order to completely stabilize the 5-hydroxy ester ⇌ 5-hydroxy acid ⇌ δ-lactone equilibrium.

3. QUANTITATIVE DETERMINATION OF PGF-M IN URINE

The method is given in detail elsewhere (1). The first step involves the addition of $[^2H_3]$ PGF-M to the urine sample and treatment with alkali. It should be emphasized that the object of the alkalinization is not to prepare the dioic acid form of the metabolite per se, but to ensure that the endogenous and ^{2}H-labeled metabolite are present in the same proportion of their dioic acid versus δ-lactone derivatives (in this case 100% dioic acid); once equilibration is achieved a fixed ratio of unlabeled to ^{2}H-labeled metabolite will be maintained during later extraction and separation procedures.

The next steps in the assay are acidification and extraction of the urine, and preparation of the methyl esters. The methylated material is then subjected to pH 10 hydrolysis. After this reaction is complete the pH 10 aqueous phase can be extracted exhaustively with organic solvent. By this means neutral and basic compounds are removed while PGF-M remains in the aqueous phase as the C-1 acid, C-16 methyl ester derivative. The sample is then acidified to pH 2, left for 1 hour at room temperature and returned to pH 8. The δ-lactone derivative of PGF-M is extracted into dichloroethane leaving almost all the urinary acids in the aqueous phase. Subsequently the metabolite is converted to the methyl ester t-BDMS ether derivative, purified further by TLC and analyzed by GC-MS.

132

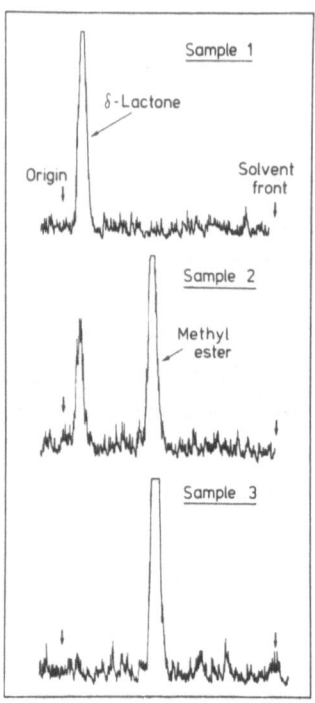

Figure 10. Thin layer radiochromatograms of the products obtained by methylation of PGF-M methyl ester δ-lactone derivative (chromatographed as their t-BDMS ether derivatives). The top trace shows the starting material. Incomplete conversion of the δ-lactone to the methyl ester was obtained when methyl iodide was added within one minute of adding methanolic TMAH and dimethylacetamide (middle trace). Quantitative conversion was achieved by treatment with methanolic TMAH for 1 hour at room temperature prior to esterification (lower trace). TLC solvent system: heptane/ethyl acetate 60/40 v/v on silica gel 60.

4. ANALYSIS OF THREE TETRANOR PGF$_{2\alpha}$ METABOLITES

The selective hydrolysis/back-extraction/methylation scheme outlined above should be applicable to the purification of other compounds which can form a δ-lactone derivative. This was tested by analysis of urine from a subject who received 60 μg of [^{2}H$_3$] PGF$_{2\alpha}$ as part of another study. Deuterium-labeled tetranor $PGF_{2\alpha}$ metabolites in the urine were measured by reverse stable isotope dilution, i.e. using unlabeled compounds as the internal standards.

To 10% of the urine collected in the first two hours following the infusion was added 400 ng each of tetranor $PGF_{1\alpha}$, 5α, 7α-dihydroxy-11-keto-tetranor (ω-dinor)-prostane-1,14-dioate (a C_{14} analog of PGF-M) and PGF-M. A duplicate urine was processed with no internal standards added. The samples were extracted, methylated and subjected to the selective hydrolysis/back-extraction/methylation sequence, essentially as described for the analysis of PGF-M itself. The TMS ether derivative was then prepared by treatment with pyridine/BSTFA. This derivative was chosen for the GC-MS analysis because a prominent ion at m/z 254 is common to the mass spectrum of the methyl ester TMS ether derivative of all tetranor $PGF_{2\alpha}$ metabolites (4,9-12). The mass spectrometer was set to record m/z 254, representing the unlabeled metabolites and m/z 257 for the corresponding deuterium-labeled compounds.

The major peak in the m/z 257 channel in Figure 11 represents deuterated PGF-M. The urine sample contained 910 ng of deuterated PGF-M per aliquot. The m/z 254 peak corresponding to PGF-M in the upper part of Figure 9 is partly accounted for by unlabeled PGF-M in the deuterated standard (m/z 254/257 = 0.1), but two thirds of the peak height is due to the normal amount of unlabeled PGF-M in urine. There was no evidence for the presence of deuterated tetranor $PGF_{1\alpha}$ in the urine (< 0.5% of the infused dose). An unidentified compound which eluted a few seconds after tetranor $PGF_{1\alpha}$ interfered with measurement of the m/z 257 peak height but selected ion monitoring of m/z 282/279 (base peak) gave a ratio which was indistinguishable from the unlabeled standard alone. About 1-2% of the infused dose was detected as the detuerated C_{14} analog of PGF-M. Granström found about four times this amount after the infusion of $PGF_{2\alpha}$ into female subjects (11).

Two aspects of this experiment deserve emphasis. Firstly, the ion current profiles are remarkably free from interfering compounds; the urinary purification procedure was sufficiently selective to enable even the endogenous (unlabeled) PGF-M to be detected with no chromatography of the samples prior to GC-MS. Secondly, the experiment demonstrates that the method can be applied to the analysis of other tetranor metabolites. n fact there are other prostaglandin-related compounds which should be amenable to purification by this procedure. These include tetranor PGD and PGE compounds (after borohydride reduc-

134

tion to their PGF analogs), tetranor thromboxane B metabolites, dinor 6-keto-PGF$_{1\alpha}$ metabolites and also 5-HETE and related fatty acids (Figure 12).

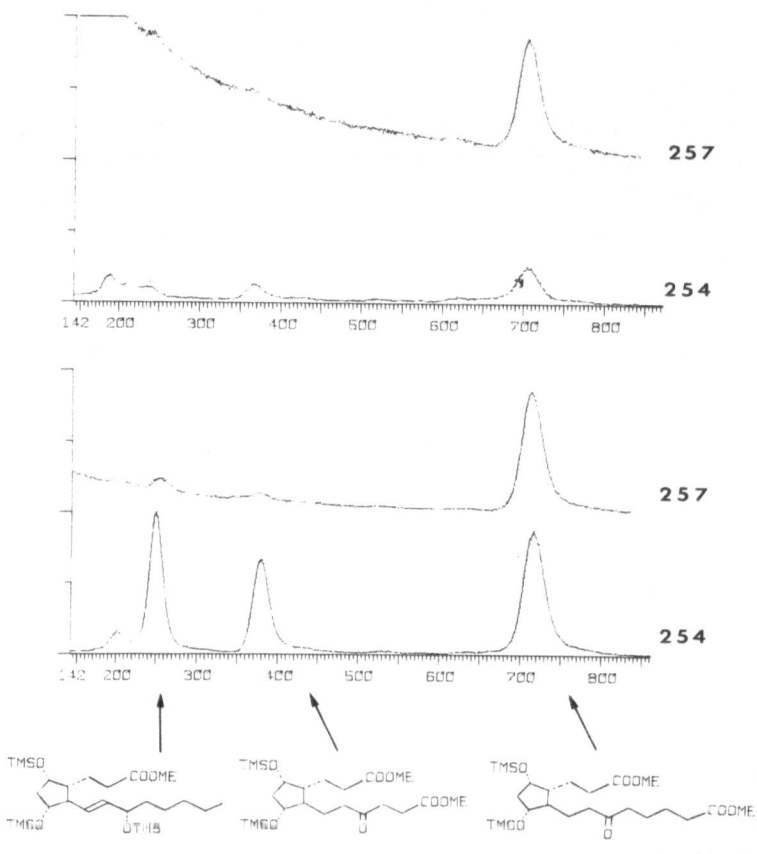

Figure 11. Analysis of urine containing deuterium-labeled PGF$_{2\alpha}$ metabolites. The upper pair of ion chromatograms correspond to the deuterium-labeled tetranor metabolites (m/z 257) and endogenous urinary metabolites (m/z 254). In the lower pair of chromatograms the three extra peaks in the m/z 254 channel represent the three internal standards added to a duplicate urine sample.

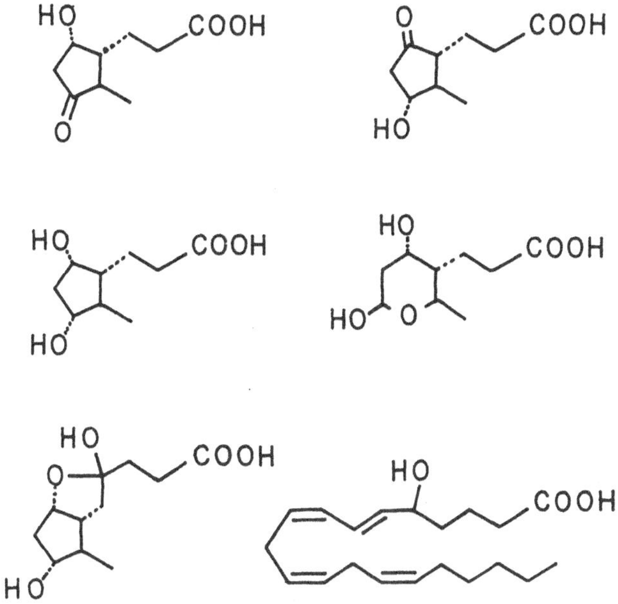

Figure 12. The basic structures of prostaglandin-related compounds which are potentially amenable to purification by interconversion of their acid and lactone forms.

5. MEASUREMENT OF PGF-M EXCRETION IN ASTHMATIC SUBJECTS

The daily excretion of PGF-M was measured in patients who were admitted to hospital with severe exacerbation of extrinsic bronchial asthma. As shown in Table I, the excretion of PGF-M in these patients was comparable to that of normal subjects (13). The Peak Expiratory Flow Rate (PEFR) values increased steadily over the course of 5 days of treatment with steroids and β-adrenergic agonists, while the PGF-M excretion remained unchanged. PGF-M is a known urinary metabolite of F, D and E series prostaglandins (9,14,15). Thus it would appear from the results in Table I that there was no elevation in the biosynthesis of F, D or E prostaglandins associated with the bronchial asthma of these particular subjects. However, one cannot completely dismiss the possibility that, for example, decreased biosynthesis of PGE was balanced by an increased production of PGF.

Table 1.   Excretion of PGF-M (ng/mg creatinine) during an asthmatic attack

Day	MALE n = 5		FEMALE n = 2	
	Excretion Rate (normal = 6.0 - 38.7)	PEFR $(l. min^{-1})$	Excretion Rate (normal = 4.6—19.0)	PEFR $(l. min^{-1})$
1	15.9 ± 6.3	131 ± 19.0	7.3 ± 1.3	98 ± 27.5
2	13.7 ± 4.3	165 ± 23.3	10.6 ± 4.5	133 ± 47.5
3	15.0 ± 4.5	195 ± 39.4	14.8 ± 6.3	158 ± 52.5
4	15.3 ± 5.2	249 ± 44.9	10.2 ± 0.1	238 ± 62.5
5	14.0 ± 4.4	338 ± 58.9	12.4 ± 1.1	360 ± 5.0

6.   EFFECT OF INDOMETHACIN ON THE BIOSYNTHESIS AND METABOLISM OF $PGF_{2\alpha}$

Four healthy male subjects received an intravenous infusion of 60 μg of $[8,10,10-^2H_3]$ $PGF_{2\alpha}$ on a control day and again one week later on the fourth day of treatment with 200 mg/day of indomethacin (16). Urine samples were collected for six hours following the infusions and analyzed for $[4,6,6-^2H_3]$ PGF-M by reverse stable isotope dilution. Urine collected during the preceding 24 hours was analyzed for endogenous PGF-M. As shown in Figure 13, indomethacin had no detectable effect on the conversion of $[^2H_3]$ $PGF_{2\alpha}$ to $[^2H_3]$ PGF-M. On the other hand the levels of endogenous PGF-M were markedly decreased by indomethacin. It can be concluded, therefore, that the decrease in endogenous PGF-M levels caused by indomethacin is due to its effect on $PGF_{2\alpha}$ biosynthesis and not to inhibition of $PGF_{2\alpha}$ metabolism.

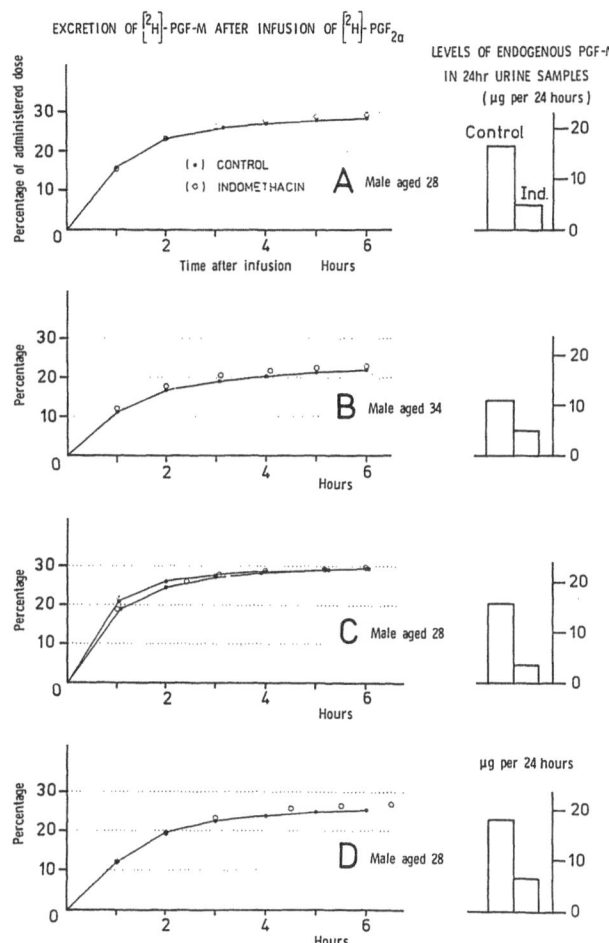

Figure 13. *Effect of indomethacin (200 mg/day) on the biosynthesis and metabolism of* PGF$_{2\alpha}$ *in man.*

7. EFFECT OF PREDNISOLONE ON THE URINARY EXCRETION OF PGF-M IN MAN

There is evidence that anti-inflammatory steroids can inhibit prostaglandin biosynthesis by the inhibition of arachidonic acid release
from phospholipid stores (17-19). It was of interest, therefore, to
examine the effects of an anti-inflammatory steroid on PGF-M excretion in man (20). Six healthy male subjects (aged 27-34) were
screened for any possible predisposition to the side-effects of anti-
inflammatory steroids. Consecutive 24 hour urines were then collected

138

before and during a course of oral prednisolone. By the last two days
of the drug treatment period, the subjects were taking a high clinical
dose of prednisolone and plasma levels of the drug confirmed compliance.

As shown in Table II, the analysis of urines from subject no. 3
was repeated. The second analysis showed an accuracy of 107% and a
precision of ± 6.7% relative to the first determination.

*Table II. Effect of prednisolone on 24 hr PGF-M excretion (μg/24 h) in
healthy male subjects.*

SUBJECT				PREDNISOLONE DOSE IN MG								
	C	C	C	15	15	30	30	60	60	C	C	C
1		15.1	16.9	12.4	13.6	17.9	15.7	21.0	16.7	21.4	15.6	
2		14.3	12.0	14.6	14.9	10.9	14.0	14.2	14.1	15.7	14.4	11.5
3	12.8	11.4	9.7	19.9	16.1	12.1	15.7	11.1	20.6	21.9	19.1	
	13.7	9.9	10.0	19.3	17.1	12.6	16.7	11.8	20.3	23.9	21.0	
4		17.6	15.9	13.0	20.2	12.0	14.7	15.5				
5		11.0	10.8	11.7	16.0	10.0	10.7	11.3	17.3	13.6	10.6	12.7
6	24.8	21.8	22.9	26.1	30.3	31.6		30.6	27.3	32.3	23.7	23.6

PGF-M output (μg/24 h) on the last day of each dose was 15.7 ±
2.1 and 14.7 ± 2.0 (control ± S.E.), 17.9 ± 1.0 (15 mg/day), 17.1 ±
3.0 (30 mg/day) and 19.2 ± 2.3 (60 mg/day). Although the mean PGF-M
excretion showed some increase with prednisolone, the increase did not
reach statistical significance. On the first day after the drug treatment period, the levels (21.0 ± 3.3 μg/day) were significantly higher
than the pre-drug values (p < 0.05, paired t test), suggesting that
prednisolone may cause an increase in PGF-M excretion in normal subjects. However it is quite certain that prednisolone did not cause a
decrease in metabolite levels in this experiment.

The results should be interpreted with caution in terms of possible effects of anti-inflammatory steroids on prostaglandin biosynthesis.
It should be noted that we do not know the tissue origin or function of

the prostaglandins which give rise to the normal levels of urinary
metabolites in animals and man. And, in most _in vitro_ experiments it
is the stimulated prostaglandin biosynthesis which has been shown to
be inhibited by steroids. It is quite possible, therefore, that both
the _in vivo_ and _in vitro_ data are valid but they simply are not monitoring comparable events. For example, one conclusion which would be
compatible with all the evidence is that the availability of free
arachidonic acid is not a rate-limiting step in $PGF_{2\alpha}$ biosynthesis in
normal subjects under 'normal' conditions. Possibly the stimulated
level of biosynthesis _is_ dependent on activation of the phospholipase
enzyme and is therefore susceptible to inhibition by steroids. Whatever
mechanistic explanations lie behind the apparent discrepancy between
the _in vivo_ and _in vitro_ results, the present experiment has established that prednisolone does not cause a decrease in the urinary excretion of PGF-M under conditions in which a substantial reduction would
be seen with indomethacin.

8. SUMMARY

The development of a GC-MS assay for the major urinary metabolite of
$PGF_{1\alpha}$ and $PGF_{2\alpha}$ is described. Two aspects of the method may have a
more general application. The synthesis of $PGF_{2\alpha}$ labeled with deuterium and tritium in the cyclopentane ring can be used for the preparation of many other prostanoic acid derivatives. And a solvent partition method for the purification of compounds which can form a lactone
circumvents some of the time-consuming LC purification steps in analysis.

It was shown that the PGF metabolite levels were not elevated in
extrinsic bronchial asthma. It was also shown that indomethacin decreased the metabolite excretion by inhibition of prostaglandin biosynthesis and not by an effect on metabolism, while prednisolone did
not reduce metabolite levels in normal subjects.

REFERENCES

1. Brash AR, Baillie TA, Clare RA, Draffan, GH: Quantitative deter-
    mination of the major urinary metabolite of prostaglandins $F_{1\alpha}$ and
    $F_{2\alpha}$ in human urine by stable isotope dilution and combined gas
    chromatography-mass spectrometry. *Biochem Med* 16: 77, 1976.

2. Nyström E, Sjövall J: Separation of prostaglandins on a hydropho-
    bic Sephadex derivative. *Anal Lett* 6: 155, 1973.

3. Brash AR, James RL: Straight-phase separation of prostaglandin
    methyl ester on lipophilic gels. *Prostaglandins* 5: 441, 1974.

4. Brash AR, Baillie TA: A comparison of t-butyldimethylsilyl ether
    derivatives for the characterization of urinary metabolites of
    prostaglandin $F_{2\alpha}$ by gas chromatography mass spectrometry. *Biomed
    Mass Spectrom* 5: 346, 1978.

5. Pike JE, Lincoln FH and Schneider WP: Prostanoic acid chemistry.
    J Org Chem 34: 3552, 1969.

6. Schneider WP, Morge RA: A synthesis of crystalline thromboxane
    B2 from a derivative of prostaglandin $F_{2\alpha}$. *Tet Lett* 3283, 1976.

7. Whittaker N: A synthesis of prostacyclin sodium salt. *Tet Lett*
    32: 2805, 1977.

8. Greeley RH: Rapid esterification for gas chromatography. *J Chrom-
    atog* 88: 229, 1974.

9. Granström E, Samuelsson B: On the metabolism of prostaglandin $F_{2\alpha}$
    in female subjects. *J Biol Chem* 246: 5254, 1971.

10. Granstrom E, Samuelsson B: On the metabolism of prostaglandin $F_{2\alpha}$
    in female subjects. II Structures of six metabolites. *J Biol Chem*
    246: 7470, 1971.

11. Granström E, Samuelsson B: On the metabolism of $PGF_{2\alpha}$ in female
    subjects. Structures of two C_{14} metabolites. *Eur J Biochem* 25:
    581, 1972.

12. Sun FF, Stafford JE: Metabolism of prostaglandin $F_{2\alpha}$ in Rhesus
    monkeys. *Biochim Biophys Acta* 369: 95, 1974.

13. Conolly ME, Brash AR, Greenacre JK: Prostaglandins in intrinsic
    bronchial asthma. *Clin Sci Mol Med* 52: 25P, 1977.

14. Hamberg M, Wilson M: Structures of new metabolites of prostaglan-
    din E_2 in man. *Adv Biosciences* 9: 39, 1974.

15. Ellis CK, Smigel MD, Oates JA, Oelz O, Sweetman BJ: Metabolism of
    prostaglandin D_2 in the monkey. *J Biol Chem* 254: 4152, 1979.

16. Brash AR, Conolly ME: The effect of indomethacin on the biosynthe-
    sis and metabolism of $PGF_{2\alpha}$ in man. *Prostaglandins* 15: 983, 1978.

17. Gryglewski RJ, Panczenko B, Korbut R, Grodzinska L, Ocetkiewicz A: Corticosteroids inhibit prostaglandin release from perfused mesenteric blood vessels of rabbit and from perfused lungs of sensitized guinea pig. *Prostaglandins* 10: 343, 1975.

18. Nÿkamp FP, Flower RJ, Moncada S, Vane JR: Partial purification of rabbit aorta contracting substance-releasing factor and inhibition of its activity by anti-inflammatory steroids. *Nature* 263: 479, 1976.

19. Tam S, Hong SL, Levine L: Relationships among the steroids of anti-inflammatory properties and inhibition of prostaglandin production and arachidonic acid release by transformed mouse fibroblasts. *J Pharm Exp Therap* 203: 162, 1977.

20. Brash AR, Conolly ME: The effect of prednisolone on the urinary excretion of the major urinary metabolite of $PGF_{2\alpha}$ in man. Submitted for publication.

DISCUSSION

M. Claeys   What is your experience making the t. butyldimethyl-silylethers at the low nanogram level ?

A. Brash   We have had some problems with this reagent in the past, but generally we can obtain good yields at the low nanogram level. It is important to recognize that the reagent is a lot less stable than BSTFA or BSA.

R. W. Kelly   The ideal way to keep this reagent is to keep 4 M solution of imidazole in dry DMF 2 M t. butyl-dimethylsilylchloride also in DMF, and add equal volumes to the extract. The temperature is also important : the reaction should be done at 120° for 1/2 hour.

9 THE MEASUREMENT OF THE UTERINE PRODUCTION OF 6-OXO-PROSTAGLANDIN $F_{1\alpha}$

R.W. Kelly, I. Cooper, S.K. Smith* and M.H. Abel*

Introduction

Several studies (1-4) have shown high concentrations of
PGE and PGF in human endometrial tissue. The concentration rises during the secretory phase of the cycle
reaching a maximum around the time of menstruation.
However, despite the findings of high concentrations of
6-oxo-PGF$_{1}$$\alpha$ (the main metabolite of PGI$_2$) in incubations
of uterus from sheep, rat and guinea-pig (5) the extent
of production of prostacyclin or its metabolites by the
human uterus is not known. A relaxing action of PGI$_2$ on
human myometrium in vitro has been reported (6) and it is
known that this compound has a marked vasodilatory action
(7) and inhibits platelet aggregation. Thus production of
PGI$_2$ by the uterus is likely to have a significant action
on blood flow within the organ. We have therefore studied
the production of PGI$_2$ by the non-pregnant human uterus
by using a GCMS technique for the measurement of 6-oxo-PGF$_{1}$$\alpha$
We have accompanied the GCMS measurements by a radiometric
assay of 6-oxo-PGF$_{1}$$\alpha$ production by both human and rat
uterus and investigated the action of catechol oestrogens
(neutral labile metabolites of oestrogens recently reviewed
in 8) on prostaglandin production by the uterus.

Materials and Methods

Prostaglandin standards. Authentic prostaglandins E_2, $F_2\alpha$, 6-oxo-PGF$_1\alpha$ and 3,3,4,4-tetradeutero PGE$_2$ were the gift of Dr. J.E. Pike and Dr. U. Axen of the Upjohn Co. 20 ethyl PGF$_2\alpha$ was the gift of Dr. N.S. Crossley, of I.C.I (Pharmaceuticals) Ltd., and 20 methyl 6-oxo-PGF$_1\alpha$ was prepared from 20-methyl PGI$_2$ which was the gift of Dr. D.A. Van Dorp of Unilever Ltd., (Vlaardingen).

GCMS Measurement of 6-oxo-PGF$_1\alpha$. Samples of endometrium were obtained at operation for a variety of non-malignant conditions. The sample was weighed and immediately placed in ice cold ethanol. The tissue was homogenised in the ethanol and centrifuged. The supernatant was evaporated and stored at $-15^{\circ}C$ to $-20^{\circ}C$ until used, whereupon it was dissolved in a fixed volume of ethanol and an aliquot was added to a fourfold excess of a solution of hydroxylamine hydrochloride (50 mg/ml) in pyridinium acetate buffer (pH 5.1, 1.5 M). Where 20-methyl-6-oxo PGF$_1\alpha$ was used as internal standard, this was added together with the extract as were 20-ethyl PGF$_2\alpha$ and 3,3,4,4-tetradeutero PGE$_2$. However when the trideutero methylester was used it was added after methylation (see below). The hydroxylamine hydrochloride solution was heated at $60^{\circ}C$ for 40 mins. and then extracted with a five fold excess of ether/ethyl acetate (3:1). The ethereal solution was washed with water and evaporated. The residue was methylated with diazometh- ane and transferred to a 50 mm x 3 mm I.D. glass tube with 50 ul of 4M imidazole and 50 ul of 2M t-Butyldimethylchlo- rosilane both dissolved in dry DMF. The tube was sealed in a flame and heated to 120° for 30 mins. The tube was broken open and the contents placed on top of a 20x5 mm column of Sephadex LH20 swollen in hexane/ethyl acetate (4:1) and washed and an aliquot injected into the GCMS in toluene. Two GCMS instruments were used in these studies a Dupont 490B coupled with a glass jet separator to a Varian 1400 GC and a VG Micromass 305F coupled through a glass jet separator to a Carlo Erba gas chromatograph. In

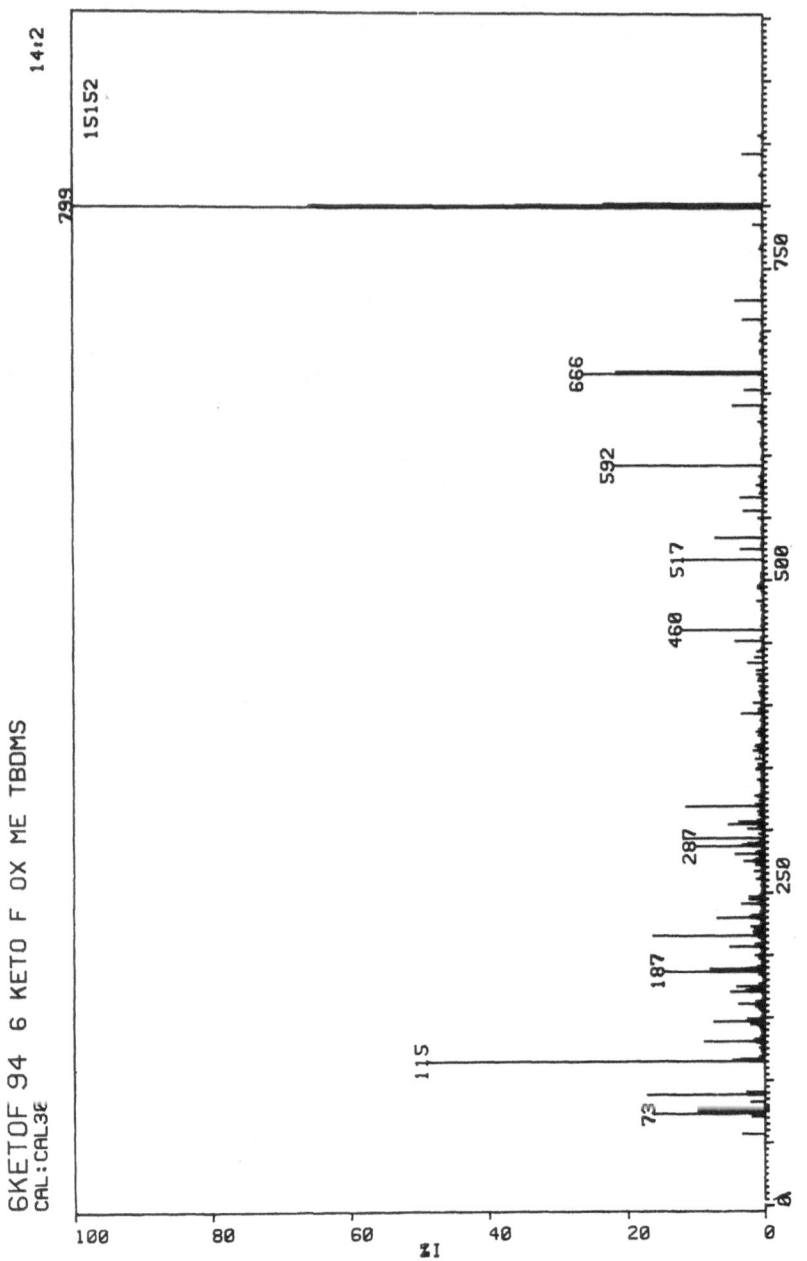

Figure 1.   Mass spectrum of 6-oxo-prostaglandin $F_{1\alpha}$ oxime, methyl ester tBDMS. M-57 is at m/e 798.54

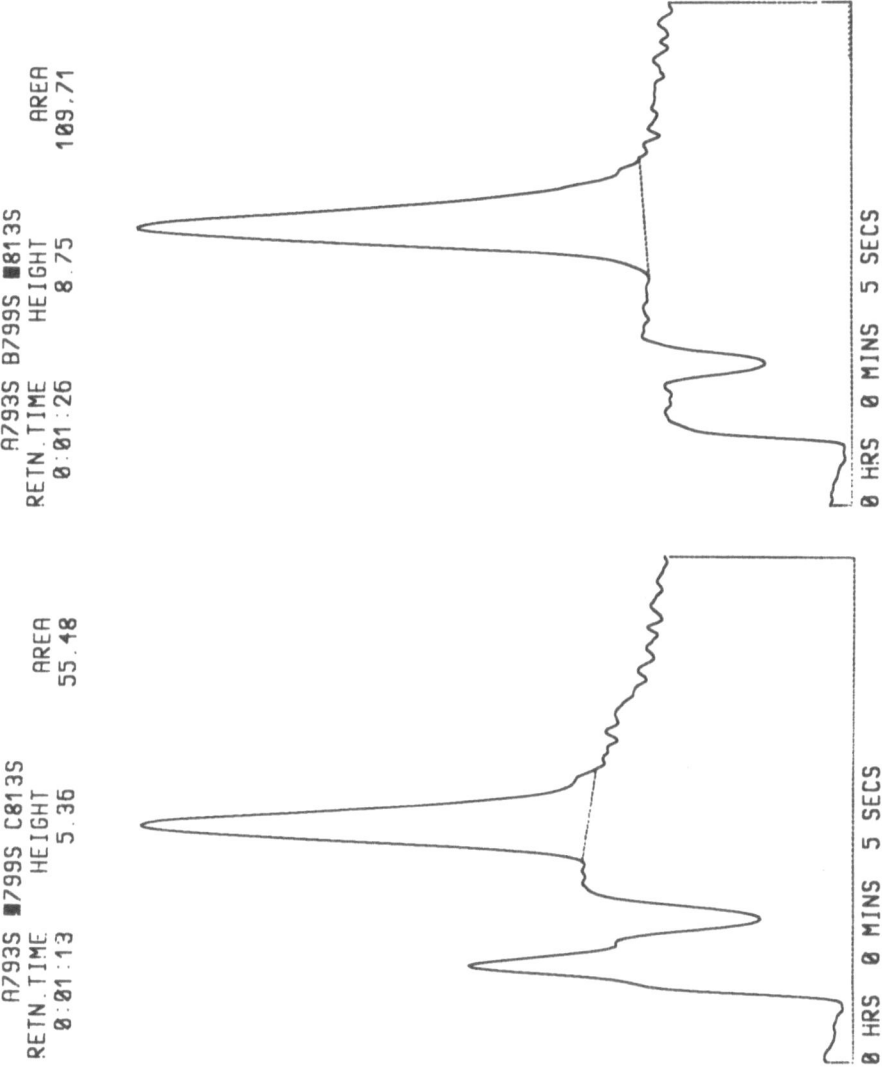

Figure 2.   Tuned ion traces of 6-oxo-PGF$_1\alpha$ (m/e 798.54) and the internal standard 20-methyl-6-oxo PGF$_1$ M/E 912.56) as the oxime, methyl ester tBDMS.   The sample is peripheral plasma (sheep) spiked with 2ng/ml of 6-oxo-PGF$_1^\alpha$(1/15 injected).

146

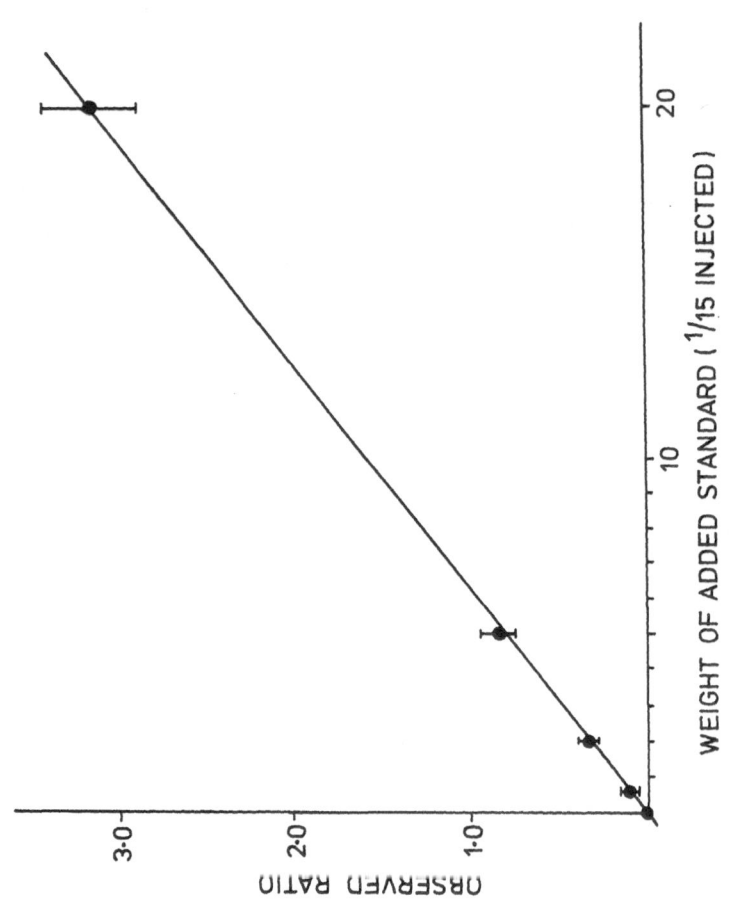

Figure 3.   A typical calibration line for the measurement of 6-oxo-PGF$_1\alpha$ using 20-methyl-6-oxo PGF$_1\alpha$ as the internal standard.

this second instrument data was recorded using the VG2150
data system. Concentrations were determined using peak
height or peak area measurements.

Results and Discussion

We have devised a method of measurement of 6-oxo-PGF$_1$
which depends on the oximation of the compound in aqueous
solution. This approach has the advantages of 1. the
reduction of the polarity of 6-oxo-PGF$_1$, allowing its
easier extraction and 2. a reliable oximation procedure
with minimum manipulation of the sample. The process of
oximation in aqueous solution seems anomalous since the
formation of an oxime involves the elimination of water,
however, the equilibrium constant K_1 for the reaction

$$\diagdown\!C{=}O + NH_2.OR \xrightleftharpoons{\quad K_1 \quad} \diagdown\!C{=}N.OR + H_2O$$

is large, and the formation of oxime is favoured. The
reaction involves general acid catalysis by a high concentration of acetate ion provided by the pyridinium acetate
buffer. The advantages of the tBDMS ether as derivative
are the concentration of a large part of the ion current
in the base peak at (M-57) and the high mass of this base
peak (Fig. 1) which is (M/e 798.5 for the oxime/methyl
ester tBDMS ether of 6-oxo PGF$_1\alpha$). The oxime rather than
the methyl oxime is used in this assay because the methyl
oxime gives significant peaks at M-31 due to the loss of
the O-Me group. The sensitivity of the measurement is
good, 30 pg of standard injected can be detected with a
signal to noise ratio of 4:1. The sensitivity of the assay
depends on the sample analysed, however 6-oxo-PGF$_1\alpha$
measured in lung perfusates at a concentration of 33 ng/ml
is measured with a relative standard deviation of 7%.
(using the trideutero methyl ester as the internal
standard).
20 methyl-6-oxo PGF$_1\alpha$ is an ideal internal standard
because of the very low contribution of the standard at
the m/e monitored to detect 6-oxo-PGF$_1\alpha$. A straight

dose response relationship is found with this standard
(see Figure 2) whereas measurements of dose/response lines
using the trideuteromethyl ester of 6-oxo-PGF$_1\alpha$ as internal
standard showed some non-linearity, due to the contribution
of 6-oxo-PGF$_1\alpha$ isotope peaks to m/e 701 monitored for
the trideutero internal standard.

We have assayed 6-oxo-PGF$_1\alpha$ in the human endometrial samples
using the trideuteromethyl ester as internal standard and
we have found undetectable or very low levels in almost all
samples. In a series of 38 samples, 6-oxo PGF was undetectable in 24 samples (limit of detection was around 100 pg
injected into the GC and because of the variable weight of
tissue available this meant a lower limit of detection
between 5 and 50 ng/gr wet weight). Of the 38 samples, 31
were below 50 ng/gr and the highest was 283 ng/g which
compares with PGE and PGF levels measured in the same
samples by a previously described method (4) which were
464 $\pm$ 655 ng/g for PGE$_2$ and 644 $\pm$ 954 ng/g for PGF$_2\alpha$.
The use of radiolabelled precursors to examine the formation of 6-oxo-PGF$_1\alpha$ (and presumably therefore prostacyclin)
is a technique which is complementary to that of GCMS. In
radiolabelled studies all extractable compounds formed
from the label appear in a thin layer chromatogram and
therefore any metabolism by alternative pathways is immediately apparent, but with GCMS the high specificity ensures
that only the chosen compound or compounds are measured.

We have used a radiolabelled technique for investigating
further the production of prostacyclin by the human uterus
(9) and have confirmed that the endometrium produced very
little. Human myometrium can only produce small quantities
of 6-oxo-PGF$_1\alpha$, (although this is the major PG produced)
but when the two tissues are incubated together there is
a relatively large production of 6-oxo-PGF$_1\alpha$ (Table 1).
We have thus shown a differential production of prostaglandins by the tissues of the human uterus although the
exact interrelationship between the tissues in vivo and
the flux of intermediates between them is at present
uncertain.

The production of prostaglandins by the uterus (among other

Table 1

Prostaglandin production by incubation of human endometrium and myometrium (mean ± S.E.M) expressed as % Arachidonic Acid converted

	6-oxo PGF$_1\alpha$	F$_2\alpha$	E$_2$	D$_2$	Total
ENDOMETRIUM n=10	0.06 ± .02	0.59 ± .20	0.77 ± .19	0.11 ± .03	1.51 ± .39
MYOMETRIUM n=6	0.19 ±	0.03 ±	0.05 ± .01	0.02 ± .01	0.29 ± .06
ENDOMETRIUM + MYOMETRIUM n=10	0.89 ± .28	0.22 ± .06	0.60 ± .22	0.12 ± .04	1.73 ± .49

organs) is regulated by steroid hormones; in particular,
there is considerable evidence that oestrogens stimulate
prostaglandin production (10). We have suggested that
catechol metabolites of oestradiol (2 or 4 hydroxy oestradiol) may be intermediates in the action of 2-hydroxy
oestradiol on PG production by the rat uterus (11) and
found that 5-250 μM concentrations of this compound markedly stimulate the production of $PGF_2\alpha$ and PGE_2 but give
a decreased production of prostacyclin (Table 2) no other
recognised co-factor of prostaglandin production such as
tryptophan or glutathione has any effect approaching that
of the catechol oestrogen. Adrenalin may have a similar
action to that of catechol oestrogen, in our experiments
it showed a small but marked action of PGF and $6\text{-oxo-PGF}_1\alpha$
production but the extent of its effect might have been
partly masked by the ready oxidation of this catecholamine
in the presence of a prostaglandin synthesising system (12).
Catechol oestrogens are also prone to oxidation (8) even in
the absence of PG generating enzymes and this may be the
reason that marked effects cannot be obtained at even lower
concentrations of these compounds. In order to test the
specificity of the effect of catechol oestrogens we have
compared the action of 2-hydroxy oestradiol with that of
its 17β - acetate, a compound similar in all respects
except in it's unnatural acetoxy group on the steroid D.
ring. We measured the production of PGF and 6-oxo-PGF by
rat uterine homogenates by GCMS and found that the 17β -
acetate at 100 μm has no effect comparable with that of the
catechol oestrogen (Table 2). We have recently found that
the action of 4-OH oestradiol (another neutral catechol
oestrogen) has a similar stimulatory action on PGF production but this is not accompanied by a decrease in
$6\text{-oxo-PGF}_1\alpha$ production as found for 2-hydroxy oestradiol
(13). In this respect 4-hydroxy oestradiol has an effect
similar to, but more potent than adrenalin.
The study of PGI_2 production by the uterus is important not
only for the reproductive aspects but also becuase local
production by the uterus argues against the concept that
PGI_2 is a circulating hormone (14, 15) we must therefore

Table 2

The effect of catechol oestrogens in prostaglandin production by rat uterus homogenates

Means $\pm$ S.E.M.

COEZYME	ng/ml $PGF_2\alpha$	ng/ml 6-oxo PGF_1	6-oxo $F_1\alpha$ /$F_2\alpha$ Ratio
CONTROL	48 ± 8.8	117 ± 20	2.4
2-OH OESTRADIOL 17	413 ± 38	82 ± 5.6	0.20
2-OH OESTRADIOL-17 ACETATE	79 ± 5.0	103 ± 3.5	1.30

use a variety of techniques to study production and metabolism of PGI_2 metabolites within the uterus. The above
studies represent the start of the measurement of the
production and excretion of these metabolites by the
uterus and hopefully will lead to eventual elucidation of
the role of PGI_2 in this organ.

References

(1)   Downie J, NL Poyser and M Wunderlich. Levels of
      prostaglandins in human endometrium during the normal
      menstrual cycle. J. Physiol 236 465, 1974.

(2)   Levitt TM, T Tobon and JB Josimovich. Prostaglandin
      content of human endometrium. Fertil Steril. 26
      296, 1975.

(3)   Singh EJ, IM Baccarini and FP Zuspan. Levels of
      prostaglandin F2 and E2 in human endometrium during
      the menstrual cycle. Am J Obstet Gynecol 121 : 1003,
      1975.

(4)   Maathuis JB and RW Kelly. Concentration of prostag-
      landins F2 and E2 in endometrium throughout the human
      menstrual cycle after the administration of clompi-
      phene or an oestrogen-progesterone pill and in early
      pregnancy. J Endocrinol 77 : 361, 1978.

(5)   Jones RL, Poyser NL and Wilson NH. Production of
      6-oxo-prostaglandin Fl by rat, guinea-pig and sheep
      uteri in vitro. Brit J Pharmacol 59, 436-437P, 1977.

(6)   Omini C, Parsargiklian R, Folco GC, Fano M and Berti
      F. Pharmacological activity of PGl2 and its metabolite
      6-oxo-PGFl on human uterus and fallopian tubes.
      Prostaglandins 15 : 1045, 1978.

(7)   Armstrong JM, Dusting, GJ, Moncada S & Vane JR. Card-
      iovascular actions of prostacyclin (PGl2), a metabolite
      or arachidonic acid which is synthesized by blood
      vessels. Circulation Res 43, I-112-I-119.

(8)   Gelbke HP, Ball P and Knuppen R, 1977. 2-hydroxy
      oestrogens, chemistry, biogenesis, metabolism and
      physiological function. In : Advances in Steroid
      biochemistry and Pharmacology Eds MH Briggs & GA
      Christie, Academic Press, NY pp 81-84.

(9)   Abel MH and Kelly RW. Differential production of
      prostaglandins within the human Uterus. Prostaglandin
      18, 821-828 (1980).

(10) Ramwell PW, Leovey EMK, and Sintetos AL. Regulation of
      the arachidonic acid cascade. Biol Reprod 16, 70-87
      1977.

(11) Kelly RW and Abel MH. Catechol oestrogens stimulate
      uterine prostaglandin production. Advances in
      Prostaglandin and thromboxane research Vol 8 Eds B
      Samuelsson, PW Ramwell and R Paoletti, Raven Press
      NY 1980 pp 1369-1370.

(12) Takeguchi C and Sih CJ. A rapid photometric assay for
      prostaglandin synthetase: application to the study in

non-steroidal anti inflammatory agents. Prostaglandin
2, 169-184, 1972.

(13) Kelly RW and Abel MH. Unpublished results.

(14) Gryglewski RJ, Korbut R and Ocetkiewicz A. Generation
of prostacyclin by lungs in vivo and it's release
into the arterial circulation. Nature 273, 765-767
(1978).

(15) Moncada S, Korbut R, Bunting S and Vane JR. Prostacyclin is a circulating hormone. Nature 273, 767-768
(1978).

10 DETERMINATION OF NANOGRAM QUANTITIES OF EICOSANOIDS AS THEIR PENTAFLUOROBENZYL DERIVATIVES BY GAS CHROMATOGRAPHY WITH ELECTRON-CAPTURE DETECTION

D.H. Nugteren, E. Christ-Hazelhof and G.H. Jouvenaz

SUMMARY

A number of methods are available to determine the products of arachidonate oxygenation at nanogram level: bioassay, radioimmunoassay and physicochemical methods. One of the latter methods, gas chromatography of suitable derivatives with electron-capture detection (GC-EC), found only limited application. However, this method has some advantages compared with for example GC-MS: the equipment needed is not very expensive and several prostaglandins can be determined in one and the same analysis. Prostaglandins of the E and A-series can be determined by GC-EC after conversion into PGB, other eicosanoids require the introduction of a special group such as bromosilyl, heptafluorobutyryl or pentafluorobenzyl. Especially the latter derivative proved to be of great value: the 5 eicosanoids PGE_2, PGD_2, $PGF_{2\alpha}$, thromboxane B_2 (TXB_2) and 6-keto-$PGF_{1\alpha}$ could be determined separately in one assay as their pentafluorobenzyl-esters or -oximes. Very reliable results were obtained when suitable internal standards with 19 or 21 carbon atoms were added at the beginning of the analysis.

The method has been applied to many biological systems: perfused heart, lung and vascular tissue, arterial and venous blood, culture fluids from various cells (from endothelium, blood, bone, thymus) and blood platelets. The influence of diet (different poly-unsaturated fatty acids, e.g. n-6 versus n-3), medicines (aspirin) and drugs (nicotine) was studied. We could not detect any prostacyclin (< 20 pg/ml) in whole human blood obtained during diagnostic catherization of the arteries and veins of the lung. So the suggestion that prostacyclin is a circulating hormone could not be confirmed. In studies with platelets and vascular tissue from rats on a cod-liver oil diet (rich in (n-3)-eicosapentaenoic acid) only negligible quantities of TXA_3 or PGI_3 were found; on the contrary, 20:5(n-3) rather inhibited the conversion of 20:4(n-6) into TXA_2 or PGI_2. On the other hand, 12-hydroxy-20:5, formed by the platelet enzyme, the arachidonate-lipoxygenase, was found in relatively large amounts.

INTRODUCTION

If one wants to determine prostaglandins at nanogram level, three different methods are recommended: bioassay, radioimmunoassay (RIA) and gas chromatography-mass spectroscopy (GC-MS). These methods will be discussed at this workshop by several investigators and the advantages and disadvantages of each of these techniques will be the subject of a debate. It is clear that having all assays available would be the most ideal situation but for practical reasons restrictions are often necessary. At our laboratory, bioassay and GC-MS are applied for various purposes and facilities and some experience with RIA are available.

The objective of this contribution is to discuss still another method for the analysis of the prostanoids and similar compounds (the "eicosanoids"), used by other investigators to a limited extent compared with the three assays mentioned above, namely gas chromatography with electron-capture detection (GC-EC).

ELECTRON-CAPTURE GAS CHROMATOGRAPHY

As early as 1970, GC-EC proved to be of great value for the analysis of the prostaglandins E (1,2). It is possible to convert PGE quantitatively into PGB with the help of alkali, and this reaction can equally well be performed when only nanograms are present in a complicated biological sample. PGB has the inherent property to display a high affinity for low energetic (thermic) electrons, because as a structural element it has a ketogroup in conjugation with two double bonds, and nanogram quantities of its derivatives are detectable with an electron-capture cell. The method we developed is depicted in Fig. 1.

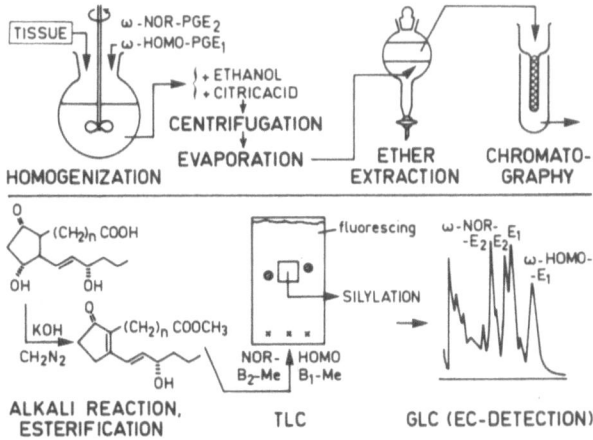

Fig. 1. Scheme for the determination of prostaglandins E by gas
chromatography with electron-capture detection.

The sample was extracted and purified on SiO_2, followed by alkali-
treatment, esterification and further purification of the PGB-ester by
TLC. Finally the silylated derivative was subjected to GC-EC. An
accurate analysis is possible when suitable internal standards (e.g.
prostaglandins with 19 or 21 carbon atoms) are added at the beginning
of the assay: in this way the losses occurring during the extraction,
purifications and chemical modifications are corrected automatically.

We demonstrated with this technique inter alia that essential fatty
acid (EFA) deficient rabbit kidney medulla and rat skin epidermis
produced less PGE_2 than animals on a normal diet. A large increase of
the PGE_2-concentration in human amniotic fluid during labour was
demonstrated. A general finding was that the standing concentration of
prostaglandins in the tissues is very low (the seminal glands of man,
ape and sheep are exceptions); the levels increase dramatically when
the intact tissue is squeezed or during homogenisation in buffer -even
at $0^\circ C$ (see Table I).

Table I

Prostaglandin E_2 content of rat epidermis

Diet	Homogenized in	ng PGE_2/g
Normal	alcohol	0 , 20
Normal	buffer	230 , 560
EFA-deficient	buffer	50

The method discussed above is not applicable to prostaglandins of the F and D series, nor could the newer members of the family - thromboxane and prostacyclin - be determined. In these cases, special groups with a high affinity for electrons (halogenides are noteworthy in this respect) must be attached to the molecules to be determined. In the steroid field, heptafluorobutyrate (HFB) and bromo-(or iodo-) methyldimethylsilyl (BMDMS) have been used for this purpose. The HFB-derivatives of the prostaglandins appeared to decompose during the conditions of GLC. We achieved some success with the BMDMS-derivatives, but the samples were not easy to analyse:especially the excess reagent gave difficulties during the EC-detection. Better results were obtained with the more recently developed pentafluoro-benzylesters and -oximes (3,4). Conversion of the oxogroup, which is present in many eicosanoids, into the oxime is advantageous for a number of reasons:

a. the oximes of PGE and PGD are stable during GLC; without derivatisation dehydration occurs (Cf. Fig. 2).

b. 6-Keto-PGF$_{1\alpha}$ consists of a mixture of open and different hemiketal forms: sometimes streaking occurs during TLC and two peaks are obtained on GLC. Similar effects can be found with TXB$_2$.

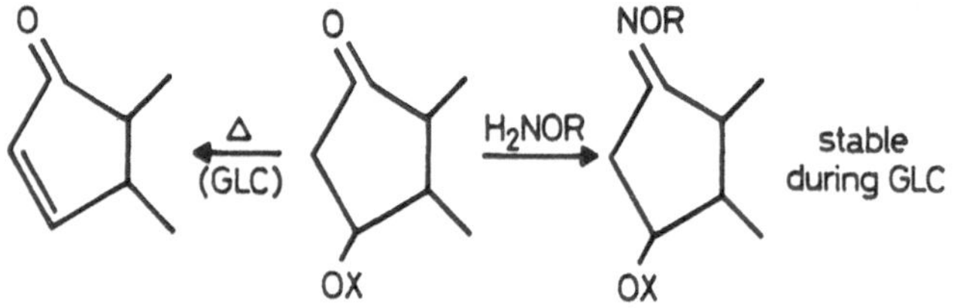

Fig. 2 Formation of the oxime of PGE or PGD.

It should be taken into account that during oxime formation a mixture of syn- and anti-isomers is formed.

PENTAFLUOROBENZYL-DERIVATIVES OF THE EICOSANOIDS

We have developed a method to determine the five eicosanoids PGE$_2$, PGD$_2$, PGF$_{2\alpha}$, TXB$_2$, and 6-keto-PGF$_{1\alpha}$ separately in one analysis as either their pentafluorobenzyl- (PFB-) esters or -oximes (Cf. Fig. 3). TXB$_2$ and 6-keto-PGF$_{1\alpha}$ are the chemically stable but biologically inactive hydrolysis products from the labile, biologically active TXA$_2$ and

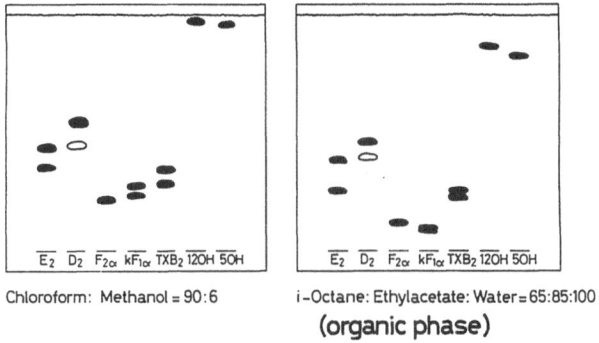

$(CH_3)_3$
Si
O

OCH_3
N

$COOCH_2$ — (F F / F / F F)

O
Si
$(CH_3)_3$

O
Si
$(CH_3)_3$

M=795

Fig. 3. Derivatized PFB-ester of 6-keto-PGF$_{1\alpha}$.

PGI$_2$ (prostacyclin). At our laboratory, very useful internal standards in the form of nor- and homo-derivatives such as ω-nor-PGE$_2$, ω-homo-PGD$_1$, ω-homo-6-keto-PGF$_{1\alpha}$, etc. are available. These have been prepared by biosynthesis and further chemical modification from the corresponding nor and homo fatty acid substrates. When known amounts of these internal standards are added at the beginning of the analysis, very reliable results can be obtained. A good example is the analysis of perfusates from isolated rat and rabbit heart which has already been described (5). After acidification to pH=3, the prostaglandins were extracted with ethylacetate, the extract dried with Na$_2$SO$_4$ and evaporated. The residue was methoximated with CH$_3$ONH$_2$.HCl after which the PFB-esters were made. These esters were purified by TLC. In Figure 4

Chloroform: Methanol = 90:6

i-Octane: Ethylacetate: Water=65:85:100
(organic phase)

Fig. 4. Thin-layer chromatography of the methoximated PFB-esters of four different prostaglandins, thromboxane and two hydroxy-eicosatetraenoic acids.

the results with model compounds in two different solvent systems are given. The bands can be scraped off and, after silylation, the samples are ready for GLC-EC. A relatively large amount of 6-keto-PGF$_{1\alpha}$ was found in the perfusates of the heart (5). Further applications of this method are illustrated below where we describe our results in connection with two recent subjects, which attracted a good deal of publicity, namely the concept of prostacyclin as a circulating hormone and the possible benificial effects of n-3 fatty acids in thrombotic diseases.

PROSTACYCLIN AS A CIRCULATING HORMONE

In 2 articles in Nature (6,7) it is suggested that PGI$_2$ is constantly released from the lung and is present in arterial blood in a concentration estimated to be about 100-200 pg/ml. In addition it is suggested that the lung can be regarded as an endocrine organ and PGI$_2$ as a circulating hormone. This concept was deduced from experiments in which the deposition of platelets on a tendon strip was monitored when superfused with arterial and venous blood.

We had the opportunity to analyse whole human blood obtained directly via a catheter from the lung arteries and veins. The blood samples were from heparinised patients which underwent a diagnostic study for heart function and performance. We preferred to analyse whole blood rather than plasma in order to include in our assay also the PGI$_2$ possibly bound to receptors of the formed elements of the blood (especially of the platelets but even the erythrocytes have been reported to bind prostacyclin). The blood (10 ml) was immediately collected in 20 ml ethylalcohol in which 10 ng ω-homo-6keto-PGF$_{1\alpha}$ was present as an internal standard. The samples were kept at -20°C until analysis. 0.1 M Citric acid (10 ml) and CH$_2$Cl$_2$ (50 ml) were added while shaking and the methylenechloride layer was worked up further. After a rather extensive and time-consuming purification, we finally obtained the silylated methyl-esters of PFB-oxime in a sufficiently pure state for electron-capture GLC. The results given in Figure 5 indicate that the internal standard was recovered satisfactorily: the characteristic double peak of the syn- and anti-isomers is seen at the right R$_t$, but there is no indication whatsoever that 6-keto-PGF$_{1\alpha}$ itself is present as degradation product of prostacyclin. We conclude that under the above conditions human lung does not secrete significant quantities of PGI$_2$ in the circulation; at least less than 20 pg/ml. Our method was checked by addition of a small quantity of PGI$_2$ to blood: this addition was fully recovered and shown as a 6-keto-PGF$_{1\alpha}$ double peak on our GLC-tracings.

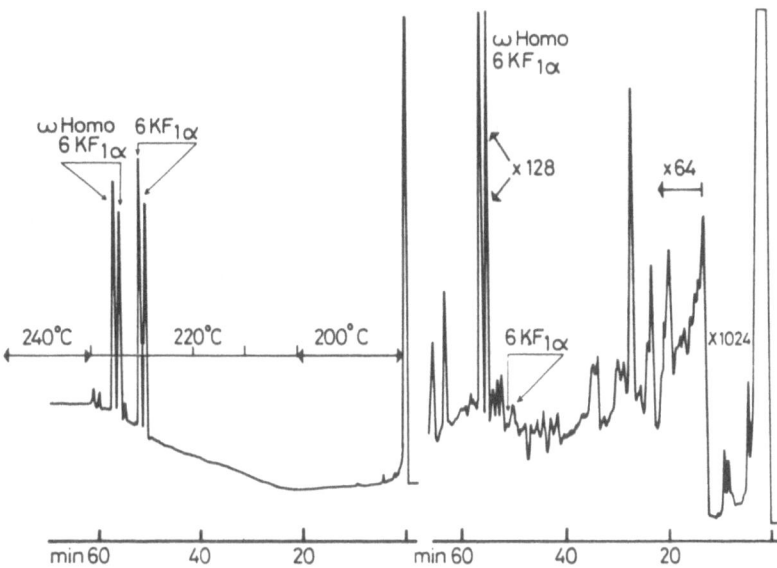

Fig. 5. Human blood studied for the presence of prostacyclin by electron-capture gas chromatography on a capillary column (SE 30; programmed from 200-240°C). Right: blood with w-homo-6-keto-PGF$_{1\alpha}$ added; left: standards.

(n-3)-EICOSAPENTAENOIC ACID IN THE DIET

Favourable effects have been reported of an Eskimo diet, rich in eicosapentaenoic acid, 20:5(n-3), on cardiovascular diseases (8). In an attempt to explain this, the aggregation of platelets under the influence of fatty acids was studied and it was found that, unlike 20:4(n-6), 20:5(n-3) did not induce aggregation in human platelet-rich plasma (see also Ref. 9). On the other hand, addition of 20:5 to a suspension of vascular tissue has been reported to result in a strong antiaggregatory activity, and this was suggested to be caused by the formation of PGI$_3$, which is of equal potency as PGI$_2$ as an inhibitor of platelet aggregation. The benificial effect of the fish oil diet of Eskimos was thus explained by a shift of the balance between the proaggregatory thromboxane and the antiaggregatory prostacyclin in favor of the latter.

PGE$_3$ and PGF$_{3\alpha}$, together with PGE$_1$, PGE$_2$, PGF$_{2\alpha}$ and PGF$_{2\alpha}$, are considered as "primary" prostaglandins and their structures were elucidated as early as the beginning of the sixties. However, it soon became apparent that the major prostaglandins in almost every animal tissue are of the 2-series, which corresponds with arachidonic acid being as a rule the major precursor. We found in experiments in vitro, using sheep vesicular gland microsomes, that 20:5(n-3) was converted only slowly and in poor yield into PGE_3, contrary to the rapid transformation of 20:3 and 20:4 into PGE_1 and PGE_2 (10). Even in tissues containing a relatively large amount of 20:5 such as the gills of fish, mussels and lobster, almost exclusively prostaglandins of the 2-series were detected (11). The (n-3)-fatty acids appeared to inhibit the conversion of the better (n-6)-substrates (12).

We have studied vascular tissue and platelets of rats on a diet with much sunflower seed oil (SO), rich in linoleic acid (18:2) the precursor of 20:4, and compared the results with those obtained from rats on cod-liver oil (CLO) with much 20:5. The SO-rats had a normal amount of 20:4 in their phospholipids but in the CLO-rats about half of the 20:4 had been replaced by 20:5.

We measured the PGI_2 and PGI_3 production in pieces of aortas of rats on these 2 diets, using the PFB-oximes, again with ω-homo-6-keto-$PGF_{1\alpha}$ as internal standard. The procedures were checked with synthetic Δ17-6-keto-$PGF_{1\alpha}$. This hydrolysis product of PGI_3 could not be detected in the samples and the amount of 6-keto-$PGF_{1\alpha}$ formed was reduced in the CLO-group (see Table II).

Table II

Prostacyclin production by rat vascular tissue

Dietary fat (50 Joule %)	ng/piece of aorta (Mean ± S.D.; n=6)	
	6-keto-$PGF_{1\alpha}$	Δ17-6keto-$PGF_{1\alpha}$
sunflower seed oil	5.9 ± 2.1	< 0.?
codliver oil	2.9 ± 2.0	< 0.2

We also measured the formation of products during collagen-induced platelet aggregation in these 2 groups and it was found that the CLO-group showed decreased formation of 12-OH-17:3 (HHT) with hardly any 12-OH-17:4 detectable, indicating an inhibition of TXA_2-biosynthesis and negligible TXA_3-formation. On the other hand, the products of the lipoxygenase pathway were formed in appreciable amounts and a mixture of 12-OH-20:4 (HETE) and 12-OH-20:5 was obtained. To separate and determine these 4 hydroxy acids, HPLC proved to be a more powerful technique than GC-MS. This is illustrated in Figure 6 where results are given after collagen-induced aggregation of platelets of CLO-rats: with HPLC, added $[D_8]$-12-OH-20:4 can even be separated from endogenous 12-OH-20:4.

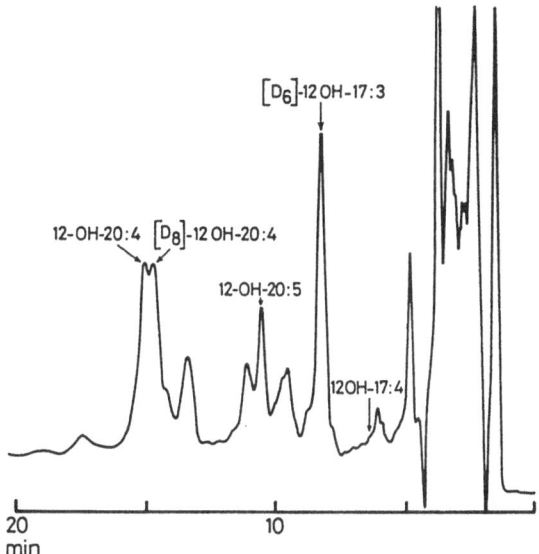

Fig. 6. High-performance liquid chromatography of conjugated hydroxy-fatty acids formed by platelets of rats on a fish oil diet (deuterated internal standards added).

Seminal fluid of a human subject on a fish oil diet was also investigated. Again, only small quantities of PG's and 19-hydroxy-PG's of the 3-series were detected, and the amount of products from the 1-and 2-series was reduced.

We conclude that so far eicosapentaenoic acid has proved to be a very poor substrate for the prostaglandin endoperoxide synthetase (cyclooxygenase + peroxidase) in every species or organ tested, irrespective of whether this enzyme is connected with prostaglandin-, thromboxane- or prostacyclin-biosynthesis.

REFERENCES

1. Jouvenaz, G.H., Nugteren, D.H., Beerthuis, R.K., and Van Dorp, D.A., Biochim. Biophys. Acta 202, 231-234, 1970.
2. Jouvenaz, G.H., Nugteren, D.H., and Van Dorp, D.A., Prostaglandins 3, 175-187, 1973.
3. Wickramasinghe, A.J.F., and Shaw, R.S., Biochem. J. 141, 179-187, 1974.
4. Fitzpatrick, F.A., Wynalda, M.A., and Kaiser, D.G., Anal. Chem. 49, 1032-1035, 1977.
5. De Deckere, E.A.M., Nugteren, D.H., and Ten Hoor, F., Nature 268, 160-163, 1977.
6. Gryglewski, R.J., Korbut, R., and Ocetkiewicz, A., Nature 273, 765-767, 1978.
7. Moncada, S., Korbut, R., Bunting, S., and Vane, J.R., Nature 273, 767-768, 1978.
8. Dyerberg, J., Bang, H.O., Stoffersen, E., Moncada, S., and Vane, J.R., Lancet, 15 July, 117-119, 1978.
9. Silver, M.J., Smith, J.B., Ingerman, C.M., and Kocsis, J.J. Prostaglandins 4, 863-875, 1973.
10. Struijk, C.B., Beerthuis, R.K., Pabon, H.J.J., and Van Dorp, D.A., Rec. Trav. Chim. 85, 1233-1250, 1966.
11. Christ, E.J., and Van Dorp, D.A., Biochim. Biophys. Acta 270, 537-545, 1972.
12. Nugteren, D.H., Biochim. Biophys. Acta 210, 171-176, 1970.

DISCUSSION

J. Frölich   With respect to the levels of circulating PGI_2 I would like to report the following observations. ^3H-6-Keto-$PGF_{1\alpha}$ -infusion in man results in the urinary excretion of this prostaglandin in unchanged form. This is in striking contrast to PGE_2, where none of the infused material was recovered in unchanged form.

Measurement of basal excretion rate of 6-keto-$PGF_{1\alpha}$ in the urine shows considerable species differences with man marking the low end of the spectrum and levels of less than 200 pg/ml. These observations would indicate extremely low levels of 6-keto-$PGF_{1\alpha}$ in the circulation. If PGI_2 should be converted to 6-keto-$PGF_{1\alpha}$ its levels would be expected to be very low.

DISCUSSION

H.W.Seyberth   1. What is the dynamic range of the linearity of the standard curve with GC-EC?

2. Don't you think that there may be quite a few peaks which interfere in the PG-analysis in quite dirty samples, such as urine (40 ml!) when using GC-EC?

D.H. Nugteren   1. We have made standard curves by injecting 50 up till 12 000 picograms pentafluorobenzyl-ester or -oxime into the gas chromatograph. Within this range, the response was linear.

2. As a matter of fact, urine contains a great many compounds and certainly the EC-method is not always specific enough to cope with such a sample. An example of the successful use of GC-EC is the determination of a characteristic urinary metabolite of PGE_2 in the rat, viz. tetranor-PGB_1, see K. Gréen and B. Samuelsson (1971) Eur. J. Biochem. 22, 391.

J.A. Salmon   You have only shown that 6-keto-PGF$_{1\alpha}$ was not detecta-
               ble in arterial blood to the lung; was there any present in
               venous blood?

D. H. Nugteren   In human arterial blood (going to the lung) as well as in
                 venous blood (leaving the lung) no 6-keto-PGF$_{1\alpha}$ could
                 be detected: the concentration must be less than 20 pg/ml
                 whole blood.

F. Dray   Are you sure that all prostacyclin is transformed into 6-keto-
           derivative when you add EtOH?

D.H. Nugteren   In one experiment we added 10 ng prostacyclin to a mixture
                 of 10 ml whole blood and 20 ml ethanol and then determi-
                 ned the recovery of 6-keto-PGF$_{1\alpha}$ using 10 ng ω-homo-
                 PGF$_{1\alpha}$ as internal standard. It appeared that the added
                 prostacyclin had been quantitatively converted into 6-keto-
                 PGF$_{1\alpha}$ during the working-up procedure.

P. Lijnen   1.   What is the average ratio of prostaglandins E$_1$, E$_2$ and E$_3$
                 in the blood of the West European?
            2.   Can you also give the average ratio of the fatty acids in
                 West European.

D.H. Nugteren   1. The concentration of prostaglandins of the E Series in
                   the blood is very low and is not detectable with most
                   assays.

                2. The fatty acid composition of blood lipids depends on
                   the diet. Normally, much arachidonic acid and only
                   small quantities of dihomo-γ-linolenic acid are present
                   (ratio about 10:1). In the case of a fish oil diet, the
                   amount of eicosapentaenoic acid can be increased con-
                   sidarably.

11 PREPARATION, PURIFICATION, CHARACTERIZATION AND ASSAY OF HYDROXY- AND HYDROPEROXY EICOSATETRAENOIC ACIDS

J.M. Boeynaems and W.C. Hubbard

PRESENCE AND ACTION OF HETES AND HPETES IN MAMMALIAN CELLS

There is growing interest in the potential biological functions of hydroperoxy-eicosatetraenoic acids (HPETEs) and hydroxy-eicosatetraenoic acids (HETEs). Transformation of arachidonic acid to one or several positional isomers of HETE has been characterized in an increasing number of mammalian tissues. Human platelets produce 12-HETE[1,2] guinea pig lung 12-, 15- and 11-HETEs[3] rabbit polymorphonuclear leukocytes 5-HETE[4], human epidermis[5] and guinea pig spleen[6] 12-HETE, rat mast cells[7] and the VX$_2$-carcinoma[8] 11- and 15-HETEs, human neutrophils 5-, 12-, 15-, 8- and 9-HETEs[9,10], human lymphocytes 5- and 12-HETEs[11] rabbit pleura, pericardium and peritoneum 12-HETE[12]. Initial reports in the literature indicate that HPETEs and HETEs have quite diverse biological activities. HPETEs modulate the activity of several enzymes. 12-HPETE inhibits platelet thromboxane synthetase[13]. 12- and 15-HPETEs block prostacyclin synthetase[14,15]. 12-HPETE inhibits platelet cyclooxygenase, stimulates its own synthesis by platelet lipoxygenase and prevents the aggregration of platelets[16]. 15-HPETE potently activates a purified preparation of cyclooxygenase[17]. 12- and 15-HPETEs activate spleen guanylate cyclase[18]. 15-HPETE enhances the release of anaphylactic mediators from the guinea pig lung[19]. In contrast with these actions which are not reproduced by the corresponding HETEs, several functions of leukocytes appear to be regulated by the HETEs themselves. 12-HETE was first shown to exert a chemotactic action upon human polymorphonuclear leukocytes[20,21]. All HETEs, except the 15-isomer, exert this action with 5-HETE being the most potent[22]. HETEs also stimulate the random migration of leukocytes and enhance the expression of receptors for complement. The chemotactic response to HETEs is specifically and competitively inhibited by HETE-methyl esters[23]. In addition to these direct observations of HPETEs

This work was supported by NIH grant GM 15431. J.M. Boeynaems is Fellow of the Fogarty International Center and Aspirant of the Fonds National de la Recherche Scientifique (Belgium). We are grateful to Dr. D. Taber for helpful suggestions.

and HETEs actions, indirect pharmacological experiments, showing stimulatory effects of arachidonic acid which are blocked by the lipoxygenase inhibitor eicosatetraynoic acid (ETYA)[24,25] but are unaffected by
low concentrations of the cyclooxygenase inhibitor indomethacin, suggest that HETEs or HPETEs could be involved in several cellular processes such as: lysosomal enzymes release by neutrophils[26,27], oxygen
metabolism in neutrophils[27], histamine secretion by mast cells[28], lymphocyte mitogenesis[29,30] and protein iodination in the thyroid[31].
Finally, the recent characterization of the structure of a slow-reacting substance produced by a murine mastocytoma as a 6-thioether-5-
hydroxy-7,9,11,14-eicosatetraenoic acid led to the hypothesis that 5-
HPETE is a precursor of this important class of mediators of allergic
diseases[32].

PREPARATION OF HYDROPEROXY- AND HYDROXY-EICOSATETRAENOIC ACIDS

Progress in the understanding of the biological functions of HETEs and
HPETEs requires the availability of large quantities of highly purified
compounds in order to test their activity. Most of the studies of the
biological activity of HPETEs or HETEs were restricted to the 12- and
15-isomers which could be prepared biosynthetically: human platelets
generate 12-HPETE or 12-HETE from arachidonic acid[13,15,17,19,20]; soy-
bean lipoxidase preparations convert arachidonic acid to 15-HPETE[33,14,
15,17,18]. A method of total chemical synthesis is not yet available
for each of the HETEs. Such a procedure was recently developed in the
case of 11-HETE (N. Nelson, personal communication). Corey and coworkers have described selective intramolecular epoxidation techniques
to generate 5,6-epoxy-8,11-14-eicosatrienoic acid and 14,15-epoxy-5,
8,11-eicosatrienoic acid[34]. These compounds can then be converted to
5-HETE and 15-HETE, respectively. Porter and coworkers have reported
the conversion of arachidonate to a mixture of HPETEs by using a photo-
chemical reaction involving singlet oxygen[35]. However, the practical
usefulness of this method was limited since the singlet oxygen reaction
also generated 6- and 14-HPETEs-compounds containing no conjugated
diene-which could not be resolved from the 5- and 15-isomers, respectively. The simple exposure of arachidonic acid to air for 72 hours
generated a mixture of 5-,8-,9-,11-,12- and 15-HPETEs[36]. The efficiency of this procedure cannot be evaluated, since these authors did not
specify their yield. In order to prepare HPETEs and HETEs, we have

modified the procedure used by Smolen and Shohet[37] to peroxidize lipo-
somes obtained from erythrocyte lipids. Reaction of arachidonic acid
with H_2O_2 in the presence of Cu^{++} ions, as described in figure 1, generates a mixture of the 6 isomeric HPETEs which can be reduced to the
corresponding HETEs with Na BH_4. Individual HPETEs or HETEs can then
be purified by high performance liquid chromatography[38,39]. The net
yield obtained with this procedure is: 5-isomer, 1%; mixture of 8- and
9-isomers, 1%; 11-isomer, 0.7%; 12-isomer, 0.4%; 15-isomer, 1%. The
primary limiting factor of this procedure is the time required to perform HPLC purification, since only limited quantities can be injected
without overloading the columns.

   MIX:

           Arachidonic Acid: 100 μmoles
           $CuCl_2$: 50 μmoles
           H_2O_2: 1.8 mmoles
           Methanol: 10 ml
           TRIS 0.2 M, pH 8.5: 2.5 ml

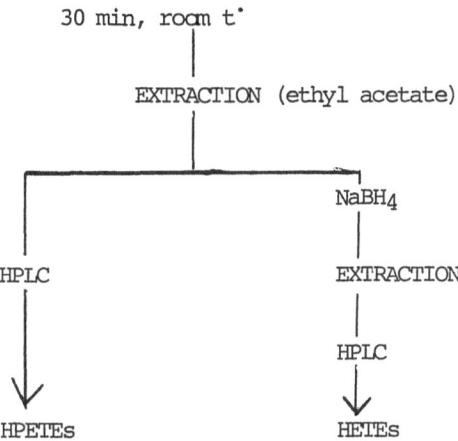

Figure 1. Preparation of HETEs and HPETEs

PURIFICATION OF HETEs AND HPETEs

HETEs can be resolved by high performance liquid chromatography. When
a mixture of HETEs is injected on a silica gel column (μ Porasil,
Waters) with delivery of a linear solvent gradient from hexane (with
0.8% acetic acid) to chloroform (with 0.8% acetic acid), the HETEs

are separated in the following sequence of elution: 12-HETE, 15-HETE, 11-HETE, unresolved mixture of 8- and 9-HETEs and 5-HETE[38] (figure 2). HPETEs can be separated in a similar way, but the recovery of 5-HPETE is very low. In order to obtain pure 5-HPETE in good yield, HPLC on a reversed phase column (μ Bondapak C_{18}, Waters) and isocratic elution with methanol-water-acetic acid (75:25:0.01, v/v) is recommended[39]. Other procedures have recently been described. 15-, 12- and 5-HETEs can be separated on a Nucleosil C_{18} column (5 μ particles, Macherey-Nagel) eluted isocratically with methanol-water-acetic acid (75:25:0.01,

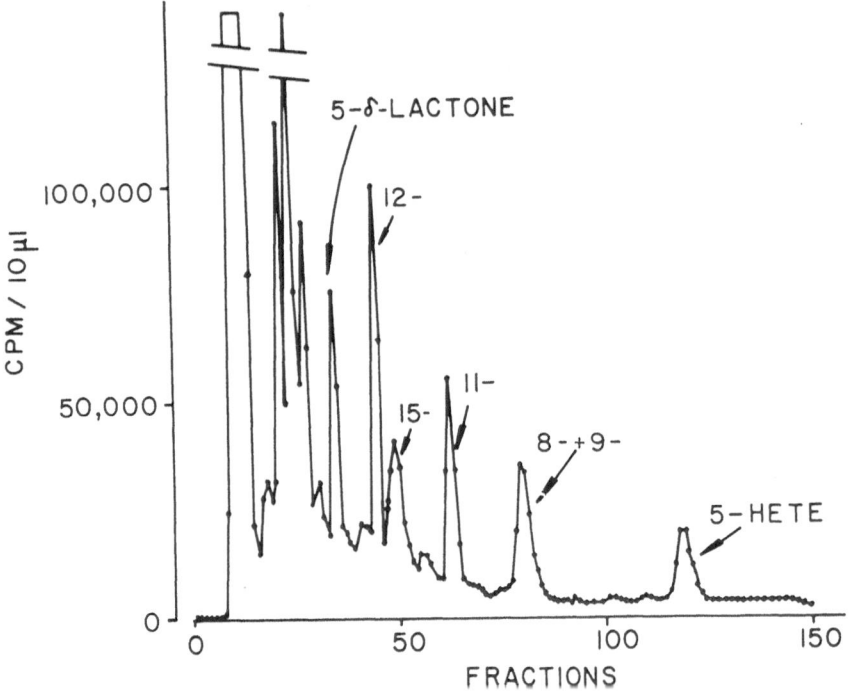

Figure 2. HPLC purification of octadeuterated HETEs. Octadeuterated arachidonate (generous gift of Dr. D. Taber), mixed with H_1^3-labeled arachidonic acid, was reacted as described in figure 1. After extraction, $NaBH_4$ reduction and a new extraction, the reaction mixture (dissolved in hexane) was submitted to HPLC on a semi-preparative column of silica gel (μ Porasil, Waters; 7.8 mm X 30 cm). A linear gradient from 25% to 65% of chloroform (with 0.8% acetic acid) in hexane (with 0.8% acetic acid) was delivered in 2 hours. The flow rate was 3 ml/m and 1.5 ml fractions were collected.

v/v)[9]. HPETEs can be separated on silica gel columns (μ Porasil, Waters) eluted isocratically with hexane-ethanol-acetic acid (993:6:1, v/v), whereas isopropanol-hexane (4:996, v/v) is suitable for the resolution of HETE-methyl esters[35,36].

CHARACTERIZATION OF HETEs and HPETEs

The HETEs and HPETEs produced by the reaction between arachidonic acid, Cu^{++} and H_2O_2 are indistinguishable from the compounds of biological origin, except for the probable lack of stereochemical purity[38]. Criteria for the identification of HETEs and HPETEs include:

- Ultraviolet spectrophotometry revealing an absorption maximum at 235 nm. This indicates the existence of a conjugated diene, having a cis, trans configuration. A conjugated diene in the trans, trans configuration has an absorption maximum at 232 nm[40,36]. Molar extinction coefficients ranging from 27,000 to 30,000 have been reported[1-4,33,35,38].

- Vapor phase properties: the retention index of the methyl ester-trimethylsilyl ether derivatives of HETEs during gas liquid chromatography is 21.3 as compared to normal fatty acid methyl esters (OV-1 column)[1,3,4,8,9,38]. Resolution of the various positional isomers of HETE by gas chromatography has not been achieved so far.

- Combined gas chromatography-mass spectrometry. The fragmentation patterns of the methyl ester-trimethylsilyl ether derivatives of the native HETEs and of the saturated compounds obtained by catalytic hydrogenation are characteristic[1,3,4,8,9,10,36,38]. The major fragment ions are listed in Table I.

Table I. *List of the major fragment ions obtained in electron ionization-mass spectrometry of hydroxy-eicosatetraenoic acids and hydroxy-arachidic acids (methyl ester, trimethylsilyl ether derivatives).*

HETE	Native compounds: m/z of major ions	Hydrogenated compounds: m/z of major ions
5-	255, 203, 305	203, 313
8-	265	245, 271
9-	255	259, 257
11-	225	287, 229
12-	295	215, 301
15-	225, 335	173, 343
all HETEs	406 (M), 391, 375	399 (M-15), 383, 367

172

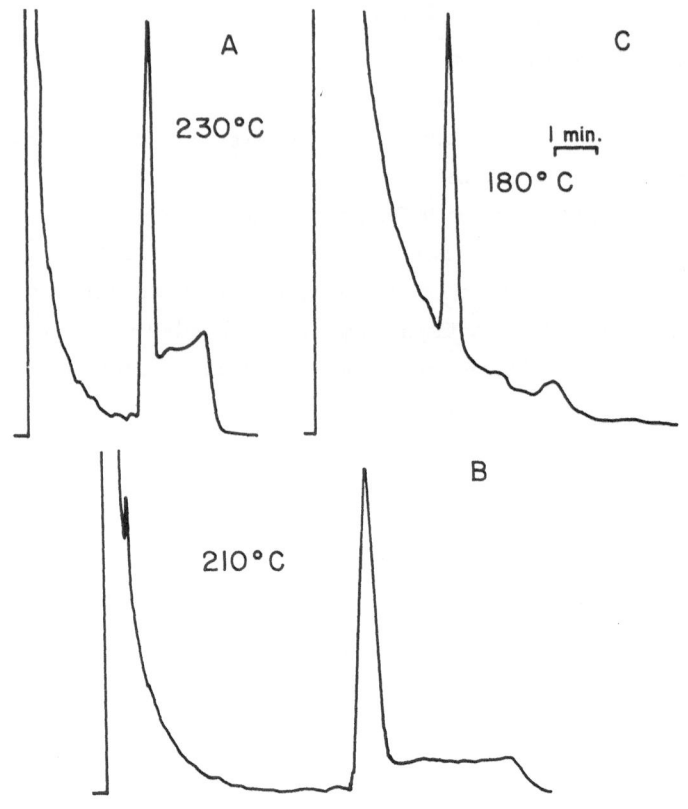

Figure 3. *Gas chromatographic behavior of 5-HETE-methyl ester-tri-methylsilyl ether at different temperatures (flame ionization detection).*

A. *3% OV-1 column (2 m X 2 mm) at 230°C; injector temperature: 275°C.*

B. *3% OV-1 column (2 m X 2 mm) at 210°C; injector temperature: 250°C.*

C. *1% OV-1 column (1 m X 2 mm) at 180°C; injector temperature: 250°C.*

5-, 12- and 15- HETEs exhibit a special behavior in gas chromatography. At column temperatures higher than 200°C, the main peak is
followed by a polydisperse tail (figure 3). The ratio between the area
of the main peak and the area of the tail decreases with increasing
temperatures. This feature is independent of the type of GC column
(OV-1 or OV-17) and of the nature of the alcool function derivatization
(trimethylsilyl ether or t-butyl-dimethylsilyl ether). This tailing
at high temperature is not observed with hydroxy-octadecadienoic acids
derived from linoleic acid or with 11-HETE. The reason for such a
difference in the thermal stability of these compounds has not been
elucidated.

The presence of a chromophore at 235 nm and the GC-MS behavior of
reduction products do not provide a tool to discriminate between HETEs
and HPETEs. The ability of peroxides to oxidize triphenylphosphine to
triphenylphosphine oxide offers a simple criterion for the differen-
tiation between HETEs and HPETEs and an easy procedure for the assay
of lipid peroxides[39]. Triphenylphosphine and triphenylphosphine oxide
can be separated by gas chromatography: equivalent chain lengths C-
18.4 and C-21.5, respectively (OV-1). A distinct advantage of this
assay over the classical spectrophotometric assays of lipid peroxides
[41,42] is the 1:1 stoichiometric relationship between the quantity
measured and the amount of peroxide added. As with other peroxide
assays, it is essential to avoid exposure of the samples to air, in
order to obtain a low blank. HPETEs are reasonably stable: when they
are stored in methylene chloride at -20°C, no loss of peroxide can be
detected for periods up to four months[39].

ASSAY OF HETEs

An assay of 5-, 12- and 15-HETEs relying on HPLC purification and UV
detection at 235 nm has been applied to human neutrophils[9]. Stable
isotope dilution assays using gas chromatography-mass spectrometry are
potentially much more sensitive. Such an assay has been developed for
12-HETE, using a deuterated standard generated by human platelets[43].
Deuterated analogs of HETEs can be prepared by a reaction beween octadeuterated arachidonic acid, Cu^{++} ions and H_2O_2[38]. Deuterated analogs
of 5-, 11- and 15-HETEs prepared by this chemical procedure are suitable for use as internal standards in stable isotope dilution assays
employing gas chromatography-mass spectrometry with selected ion monitoring. Using methyl ester trimethylsilyl ether derivatives, blanks

are less than 0.6%, linear standard curves are obtained with the injection of 100 ng of standard and the detection limit is less than 1 ng[38] (Table II).

Table II. GC-MS assay of HETEs (methyl ester trimethylsilyl ether derivatives)

	Ions monitored (m/z)	Blank (parts per thousand)	Detection Limit
5-HETE	305,313	5.9	500 pg
11-HETE	225,229	1.6	100 pg
15-HETE	335,343	3.1	400 pg

Extraction of HETEs requires less polar solvents and less acidic pH than the extraction of prostaglandins and thromboxane (figure 4). This property could be used as an easy initial purification step of samples. Further sample work-up will probably involve HPLC purification, as described earlier. The specificity of the GC-MS assay could be increased by using derivatives providing ions of higher mass, such as pentafluorobenzyl ester-trimethylsilyl ether or methyl ester-t-butyldimethylsilyl ether derivatives[44] (figure 5). However, the decreased volatility of these derivatives requires the use of higher temperatures, at which the thermolability of HETEs might be responsible for a loss of sensitivity. The potential usefulness of chemical ionization, chemical ionization with negative ion detection and capillary columns for the assay of HETEs remains to be investigated.

CONCLUSION

Multi-milligram quantities of HPETEs and HETEs can be easily generated by a reaction between arachidonic acid, Cu^{++} ions and H_2O_2 and purified by high performance liquid chromatography. Octadeuterated analogs prepared by this procedure are suitable for use as internal standards in assays by gas chromatography-mass spectrometry.

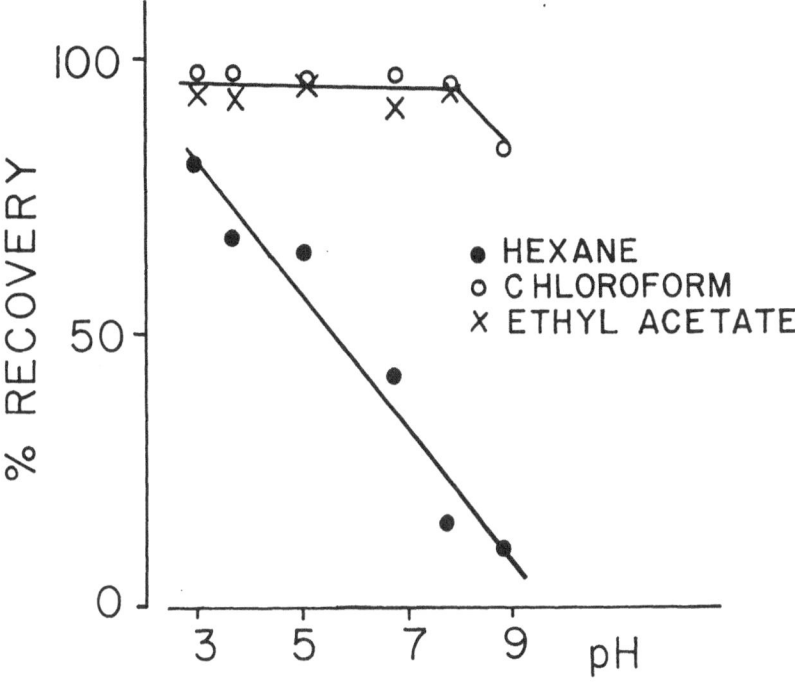

Figure 4. Extraction of 5-HETE with various solvents at various pH.
About 20 ng of D₈-5-HETE was dissolved in a modified Krebs-Ringer medium containing 20 mM Hepes, pH 7.4. After acidification with HCl 0.1N or alkalinization with NaOH 1N, two volumes of either hexane, chloroform or ethyl acetate were added. The extraction efficiency was monitored by liquid scintillation counting of radioactivity. Extraction of 5-HETE from human plasma can be performed in the same conditions.

176

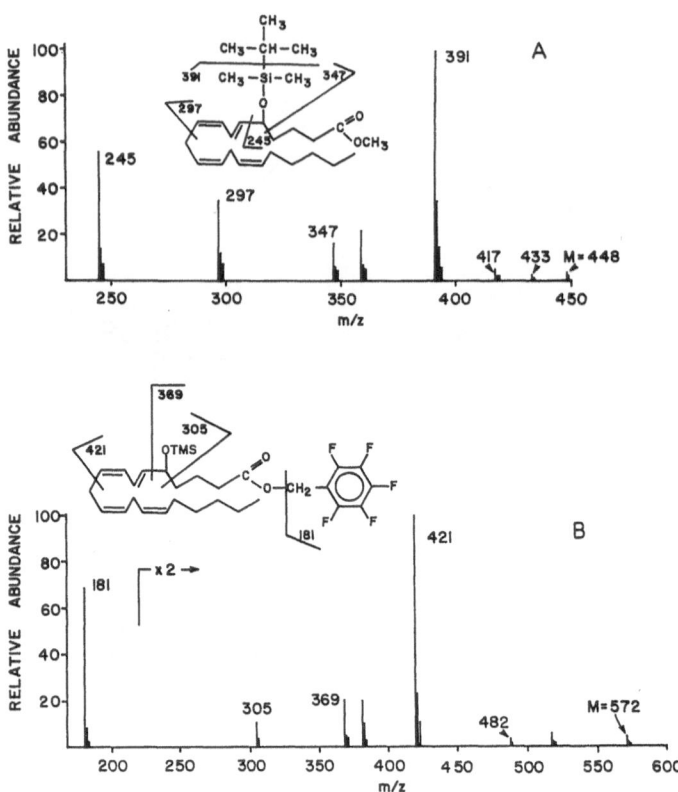

Figure 5. Mass spectra of 5-HETE-methyl ester-t-butyldimethylsilyl ether (panel A) and 5-HETE-pentafluorobenzyl ester-trimethylsilyl ether (panel B). Derivatizations were performed as described[44,45]. Mass spectra were recorded on a Hewlett-Packard combined gas chromatograph-quadrupole mass spectrometer (model 5982A). Samples were injected on a 1 m X 2 mm column of 3% OV-1 on Gas Chrom Q with helium as carrier gas (30 ml/min). The temperature of the column was 220°C. Electron energy was 70 eV.

177

REFERENCES

1. Hamberg M and Samuelsson B: Novel transformation of arachidonic acid in human platelets. *Proc Natl Acad Sci USA* 71:3400–3404, 1974.

2. Nugteren DH: Arachidonate lipoxygenase in platelets. *Biochim Biophys Acta* 380:299–307, 1975.

3. Hamberg M and Samuelsson B: Prostaglandin endoperoxides VII novel transformations of arachidonic acid in guinea pig lung. *Biochem Biophys Res Commun* 61:942–949, 1974.

4. Borgeat P, Hamberg M and Samuelsson B: Transformation of arachidonic acid and homo-γ-linolenic acid by rabbit polymorphonuclear leukocytes. *J Biol Chem* 251:7816–7820, 1976.

5. Hammarström S, Hamberg M, Samuelsson B, Duell EA, Stawiski M and Voorhees JJ: Increased concentrations of non-esterified arachidonic acid, 12-L-HETE, PGE_2 and $PGF_{2\alpha}$ in epidermis of psoriasis. *Proc Natl Acad Sci USA* 72:5130–5134, 1975.

6. Hamberg M: On the formation of TxB_2 and 12-L-HETE in tissues of the guinea pig. *Biochim Biophys Acta* 431:651–654, 1976.

7. Roberts LJ, Lewis RA, Lawson JA, Sweetman BJ, Austen KF and Oates JA: Arachidonic acid metabolism by rat mast cells. *Prostaglandins* 15:717, 1978.

8. Hubbard WC, Hough A, Watson JT and Oates JA: Evidence for the metabolism of arachidonic acid by lipoxygenase in VX_2 carcinoma. *Prostaglandins* 15:721, 1978.

9. Borgeat P and Samuelsson B: Arachidonic acid metabolism in polymorphonuclear leukocytes: effects of ionophore A23187. *Proc Natl Acad Sci USA* 76:2148–2152, 1979.

10. Goetzl E, and Sun F: Generation of unique monohydroxyeicosatetraenoic acids from arachidonic acid by human neutrophils. *J Exp Med* 150:406–411, 1979.

178

11. Parker CW, Stenson WF, Huber MG and Kelly JP: Formation of thromboxane B_2 and hydroxyarachidonic acids in purified human lymphocytes in the presence and absence of PHA. *J Immun* 122:1572-1577, 1979.

12. Herman AG, Claeys M, Moncada S and Vane JR: Biosynthesis of PGI_2 and 12-HETE by pericardium, pleura, peritoneum and aorta of the rabbit. *Prostaglandins* 18:439-452, 1979.

13. Hammarström S and Falardeau P: Resolution of prostaglandin endoperoxide synthase and thromboxane synthase of human platelets. *Proc Natl Acad Sci USA* 74:3691-3695, 1977.

14. Moncada S, Gryglewski RJ, Bunting S and Vane JR: A lipid peroxide inhibits the enzyme in blood vessel microsomes that generates from prostaglandin endoperoxides the substance (PGX) which prevents platelet aggregation. *Prostaglandins* 12:715-737, 1976.

15. Ham EA, Egan RW, Soderman DD, Gale PH and Kuehl FA: Peroxidase-dependent deactivation of prostacyclin synthetase. *J Biol Chem* 254:2191-2194, 1979.

16. Siegel ME, McConnell RT, Abrahams SL, Porter NA and Cuatrecasas P: Regulation of arachidonate metabolism via lipoxygenase and cyclooxygenase by 12-HPETE. *Biochem Biophys Res Commun* 89:1273-1280, 1979.

17. Hemler ME, Cook HW and Lands WEM: Prostaglandin biosynthesis can be triggered by lipid peroxides. *Arch Biochem Biophys* 193:340-345, 1979.

18. Graff G, Stephenson JH, Glass DB, Haddox MK and Goldberg ND: Activation of soluble splenic guanylate cyclase by prostaglandin endoperoxides and fatty acid hydroperoxides. *J Biol Chem* 253:7662-7776, 1978.

19. Adcock JJ, Garland LJ, Moncada S and Salmon JA: Enhancement of anaphylactic mediator release from guinea pig perfused lung by fatty acid hydroperoxides. *Prostaglandins* 16:163-178, 1978.

20. Turner SR, Tainer JA and Lynn WS: Biogenesis of chemotactic molecules by the arachidonate lipoxygenase system of platelets. *Nature* 257:680-681, 1975.

21. Goetzl EJ, Woods M and Gorman RR: Stimulation of human eosinophil and neutrophil polymorphonuclear leukocyte chemotaxis and random migration by 12-HETE. *J Clin Invest* 59:179-183, 1977.

22. Goetzl EJ, Brash AR, Tauber AI, Oates JA and Hubbard WC: Modulation of human neutrophil function by monohydroxyeicosatetraenoic acids. *Immunology*, in press.

23. Goetzl EJ, Valone FH, Reinhold VN and Gorman RR: Specific inhibition of the polymorphonuclear leukocyte chemotactic response to hydroxy-fatty acid metabolites of arachidonic acid by methyl ester derivatives. *J Clin Invest* 63:1181-1186, 1979.

24. Downing DT, Ahern DG and Bachta M: Enzyme inhibition by acetylenic compounds. *Biochem Biophys Res Commun* 40:218-223, 1970.

25. Tobias LD and Hamilton JG: The effect of 5, 8, 11, 14 eicosatetraynoic acid on lipid metabolism. *Lipids* 14:181-193, 1979.

26. Naccache PH, Showell HJ, Becker EL and Sha'afi RI: Arachidonic acid induced degranulation of rabbit peritoneal neutrophils. *Biochem Biophys Res Commun* 89:292-299, 1979.

27. Bokoch GM and Reed PW: Inhibition of the neutrophil oxidative response to a chemotactic peptide by inhibitors of arachidonic acid oxygenation. *Biochem Biophys Res Commun* 90:481-487, 1979.

28. Sullivan TJ and Parker CW: Possible role of arachidonic acid and its metabolites in mediator release from rat mast cells. *J Immun* 122:431-436, 1979.

29. Kelly JP and Parker CW: Effects of arachidonic acid and other un-
     saturated fatty acids on mitogenesis in human lymphocytes. *J Im-
     mun* 122:1556-1562, 1979.

30. Kelly JP, Johnson MC and Parker CW: Effects of inhibitors of ara-
     chidonic acid metabolism on mitogenesis in human lymphocytes. *J
     Immun* 122:1563-1571, 1979.

31. Boeynaems JM, Van Sande J, Decoster C and Dumont JE: Effects of
     arachidonic acid on the thyroid gland in vitro. In: *Advances in
     Prostaglandin and Thromboxane Research*, Raven Press, in press.

32. Murphy RC, Hammarström S and Samuelsson B: Leukotriene C: a slow
     reacting substance from murine mastocytoma cells. *Proc Natl Acad
     Sci USA* 76:4275-4279, 1979.

33. Hamberg M and Samuelsson B: On the specificity of the oxygenation
     of unsaturated fatty acids   catalyzed by soybean lipoxidase.
     J Biol Chem 242:5329-5335, 1967.

34. Corey EJ, Nirva H and Falck JR: Selective epoxidation of arachi-
     donic acid and eicosatrienoic acid. *J Am Chem Soc* 101:1586-1587,
     1979.

35. Porter NA, Logan J and Kontoyiannidou V: Preparation and purifi-
     cation of arachidonic acid hydroperoxides of biological importance
     J Org Chem 44:3177-3180, 1979.

36. Porter NA, Wolf RA, Yarbro EM and Weenen H: The autoxidation of
     arachidonic acid: formation of the proposed SRS-A intermediate.
     Biochem Biophys Res Commun 89:1058-1064, 1979.

37. Smolen JE and Shohet SB: Permeability changes induced by peroxi-
     dation in liposomes prepared from human erythrocyte lipids. *J
     Lip Res* 15:273-280, 1974.

38. Boeynaems JM, Brash AR, Oates JA and Hubbard WC: Preparation and
     assay of monohydroxyeicosatetraenoic acids. *Anal Biochem*, in press.

39. Boeynaems JM, Oates JA and Hubbard WC: Preparation and character-
    ization of hydroperoxyeicosatetraenoic acids (HPETEs). *Prosta-*
    glandins, in press.

40. Chan HWS and Levett G: Autoxidation of methyl linoleate separa-
    tion and analysis of isomeric mixtures of methyl linoleate hydro-
    peroxides and methyl hydroxylinoleates. *Lipids* 12:99-104, 1977.

41. Gray JI: Measurement of lipid oxidation: a review. *J Am Oil*
    Chem Soc 55:539-546, 1978.

42. Buege JA and Aust SD: Microsomal lipid peroxidation. In: *Meth-*
    ods in Enzymology, Fleisher S and Packer L (eds), Academic Press,
    1978, L11:302-311.

43. Hamberg M, Svensson J and Samuelsson B: Prostaglandin endoperox-
    ides. A new concept concerning the mode of action and release of
    prostaglandins. *Proc Natl Acad Sci USA* 71:3824-3828, 1974.

44. Sweetman BJ, Roberts LJ, Hubbard WC, Watson JT and Oates JA: The
    use of t-butyldimethylsilyl (t-BDMS)-ether derivatives in the
    structural elucidation of metabolites of thromboxane and prosta-
    glandins using GC-MS. Proceedings of 26th Annual Conference on
    Mass Spectrometry, St. Louis, 276-278, 1978.

45. Fitzpatrick F: Gas chromatography of the prostaglandins. In:
    Methods in Prostaglandin Research, Frolich JC (ed), Raven Press,
    1978, 95-119.

12 PLATELET PROSTAGLANDINS AND RELATED COMPOUNDS IN DIABETES MELLITUS

M. Lagarde, P. Berciaud, M. Burtin, M. Soulier, B. Velardo and M. Dechavanne

ABSTRACT

Diabetic platelet-rich plasmas (PRP) exhibited an hyperaggregability to collagen and sodium arachidonate. Platelets isolated from their plasma only showed an hyperaggregability to collagen but not to sodium arachidonate. In agree with that, biosynthesis of prostaglandins and related compounds from endogenous arachidonic acid (thrombin as inducer) was increased in diabetic platelets but not the biosynthesis from exogenous arachidonate. On the other hand, half-life of thromboxane A_2 was longer in diabetic plasma than in normal one. Thus, hyperaggregability of diabetic PRP to sodium arachidonate could be partly due to the increase of half-life of thromboxane A_2.

Lastly, we tested the response of platelet aggregation to prostacyclin. Our results showed a refractoriness to prostacyclin with either PRP or isolated platelets from diabetic patients. Moreover, this finding also was seen when prostaglandin E_1 was used.

INTRODUCTION

Diabetic patients show a thrombotic tendency with an increase of platelet functions (for a review see reference 1). Prostaglandins and thromboxanes are produced during platelet activation and some of those are potent pro-aggregatory molecules (2,3). Recently, some investigators have found that diabetic platelet-rich plasmas produce more prostaglandin E-like material than normal platelets when they are

aggregated (4). Otherwise, platelets obtained from diabetic subjects
are less sensitive to the antiaggregatory effects of imidazole, a
thromboxane synthetase inhibitor (5).

In this study, we mainly investigated the part of platelet-poor plasma
in platelet reactivity and prostaglandin biosynthesis from exogenous
and endogenous arachidonic acid.

METHODS

Patients with various ages (19 to 66 years old) had not taken any drug
except for insulin. The average duration of diabetes was about 12 years.
Patients were generally free from clinically apparent vascular disease.
Among them, twelve showed background retinopathy.

Patient platelets were simultaneously investigated with normal platelets from a donor with the same age and sex.

Blood collection was done on trisodium citrate 3.8 % or ACD and platelets isolated from the ACD platelet-rich plasma (PRP) (6). Platelet
aggregation was performed according to the method of Born (7).

Standards prostaglandins, prostacyclin and thromboxane B2 were generous
gifts from Dr J.E. Pike of Upjohn, Kalamazoo. Endothelial cell microsomes used to inhibit platelet aggregation were obtained from human
umbilical cord and their inhibiting activity was completely abolished
by 15-hydroperoxy arachidonic acid or tranylcypromine.

Main end-products of exogenous arachidonic acid utilization by platelets were determined with a radiochemical technique (8).

After platelet phospholipid labelling by traces of $[^{14}C]$-arachidonic
acid $(0.4.10^{-6}M$ at 50 Ci/mole), thromboxane B2, 12-hydroxy-heptadeca-
trienoic acid (HHT) and 12-hydroxy-eicosatetraenoic acid (HETE) production under thrombin stimulation, were assayed by the same radiochemical technique (8).

The half-life of thromboxane A2 in platelet-poor plasma was determined
as described (9). Briefly, radiolabelled thromboxane A2 was generated
from human platelets as enzymatic source and immediately dived in the
studied plasma. Then, aliquots of plasma were decanted in 80 volumes
of methanol to obtain mono-o-methyl thromboxane B2 from thromboxane A2
(10). Derivatized thromboxane B2 was radiochemically assayed (8) and a
semi-logarithmic regression leads to half-life determination.

RESULTS

Minimal doses of sodium arachidonate or collagen necessary to induce
50 % of platelet aggregation were determined. When PRP was used
(table I) these doses were lower, indicating an hyperaggregability to
both inducers.

TABLE I

*Minimal doses of collagen or sodium arachidonate able to induce 50 %
of platelet aggregation in PRP.*

	Collagen (n = 16)	Sodium arachidonate (n = 29)
Control	0.32 μg/ml	0.29 mM
Diabetic	0.21 μg/ml	0.22 mM
Paired test	0.11 ± 0.14 $p < 0.01$	0.07 ± 0.08 $p < 0.001$

In contrast, only collagen-induced aggregation was increased when isolated platelets were used (table II).

TABLE II

*Minimal doses of collagen or sodium arachidonate able to induce 50 %
of platelet aggregation in isolated platelets.*

	Collagen (n = 15)	Sodium arachidonate (n = 28)
Control	0.55 μg/ml	2.05 μM
Diabetic	0.34 μg/ml	1.96 μM
Paired test	0.20 ± 0.33 $p < 0.05$	0.08 ± 0.71 N.S.

Thus, isolated platelets were hyperactive to collagen but not to sodium
arachidonate. Moreover, platelet-poor plasma induced a higher response
of platelets to arachidonate.
Utilization of exogenous arachidonate by platelets isolated from their
plasma was not modified since biosynthesis of prostaglandins and related compounds as well as incorporation of arachidonate in phospholipids
were unchanged (table III).

TABLE III

Utilization of exogenous sodium arachidonate 10 μM by isolated platelets during 4 min. (nmoles of arachidonate incorporated or transformed/10^9 platelets).

	Control	Diabetic	Paired test
Phospholipids (n = 12)	6.1	4.1	2.1 ± 4.3 N.S.
$PGF_2\alpha$ (n = 13)	0.98	1.0	0.02 ± 0.68 N.S.
PGE_2 (n = 13)	0.91	0.93	0.02 ± 0.46 N.S.
TXB_2 (n = 13)	8.1	7.2	0.9 ± 4.5 N.S.
HHT (n = 10)	3.6	4.2	0.6 ± 3.0 N.S.
HETE (n = 9)	10.9	8.2	2.6 ± 3.9 N.S.

In contrast, utilization of phospholipidic arachidonate by the same pathways (as judged by thromboxane B_2, HHT and HETE), under thrombin stimulations was higher in diabetic platelets (table IV).

TABLE IV

Biosynthesis of TXB_2, HHT and HETE from endogenous arachidonic acid after stimulation by thrombin 0.1 U/ml. Results are expressed in percentage of initial radioactivity in phospholipids.

	Control	Diabetic	Paired test
TXB_2 (n = 29)	4.8	5.5	0.6 ± 1.5 $p < 0.05$
HHT (n = 28)	0.66	0.57	0.09 ± 0.90 N.S.
HETE (n = 28)	3.8	4.4	0.6 ± 1.4 $p < 0.05$
TXB_2 + HHT + HETE (n = 27)	9.2	10.4	1.2 ± 3.0 $p < 0.05$

These data indicate an enhancement of diabetic platelet phospholipase activity whereas prostaglandin synthetase and lipoxygenase activities seem normal.

Besides, the half-life of thromboxane A_2 was considerably increased in diabetic platelet-poor plasma as compared to control (table V).

TABLE V

Half-life (Min.) of thromboxane A_2 in platelet-poor plasma.

Control (n = 9)	Diabetic (n = 12)
7.2 ± 2.9	12.5 ± 5.9
$p < 0.05$	

Lastly, diabetic platelets showed a refractoriness to prostacyclin and prostaglandin E_1 inhibition. Either in the presence of prostacyclin synthetase or prostacyclin, inhibition of collagen-induced platelet aggregation was lower in diabetics than in controls. These results were observed with PRP (table VI) as well as with isolated platelets (table VII).

TABLE VI

Percentage of inhibition of collagen-induced platelet aggregation. PRP was used. Inhibitors were preincubated 1 min.

	Control	Diabetic	Paired test
Endothelial microsomes (n = 26)	55.8	40.8	14.7 ± 36.3 p < 0.05
PGI$_2$ (n = 28)	53.6	31.3	22.2 ± 31.2 p < 0.001
PGE$_1$ (n = 6)	70.3	45.5	24.8 ± 21.6 p < 0.05

TABLE VII

Percentage of inhibition of collagen-induced platelet aggregation. Isolated platelets were used. Inhibitors were preincubated 1 min.

	Control	Diabetic	Paired test
Endothelial microsomes (n = 15)	63.0	48.7	14.3 ± 16.6 p < 0.01
PGI$_2$ (n = 19)	61.5	47.1	14.4 ± 22.6 p < 0.02

DISCUSSION

Susceptibility of diabetic platelet aggregation to arachidonate, only in the presence of the plasma, suggests the effect of a plasmatic factor to enhance diabetic platelet aggregation. This fact   agrees with other recent works which strongly suggest the formation of certain platelet reactive low molecular weight proteins in some diabetic patients (5). Our results does not indicate an increase of the formation of pro-aggregatory molecules   derived   from arachidonic acid. But, the increase of half-life of thromboxane A_2 by diabetic plasma could partly explain the hyperaggregability of diabetic PRP to arachidonate. Responsiveness of diabetic platelets to collagen (aggregation) or thrombin (prostaglandin synthesis from endogenous arachidonate) was higher and has a platelet origin. These data lead to two hypotheses ; 1 : diabetic platelets contained more phospholipidic arachidonate or 2 : induced phospholipase activity was higher in patient platelets. On the other hand, patient platelets showed a refractoriness to prostaglandins I_2 and E_1 known to inhibit platelet functions by increasing platelet cyclic AMP (11,12). Thus, a possibility should be that platelet cyclic AMP, which inhibits phospholipase activity (13), be low in diabetic platelets. These last points   agree with the second hypothesis mentioned above.

ACKNOWLEDGEMENTS

This work was supported by grant INSERM ASR N°5. We gratefully acknowledge Drs F. Berthezene and Grange for sending the patients.

REFERENCES

1. Bern MM. Platelet functions in diabetes mellitus. Diabetes. 27, 342-350, 1978.

2. Samuelsson B, Hamberg M, Malmsten C and Svensson J. The role of prostaglandin endoperoxides and thromboxanes in platelet aggregation. In : Advances in prostaglandin and thromboxane research. Samuelsson B and Paoletti R (eds). New York. Raven Press. 1976, 2, 763-766.

3. Smith JB, Ingerman CM and Silver MJ. Effects of arachidonic acid and some of its metabolites on platelets. In : Prostaglandins in hematology. Silver MJ, Smith JB and Kocsis JJ (eds). New York. Spectrum Publications. 1977, 155

4. Halushka PV, Lurie D and Colwell JA. Increased synthesis of prostaglandin E-like material by platelets from patients with diabetes
   mellitus. New. Engl. J. Med. 297, 1306-1310, 1977.

5. Colwell JA, Nair RMG, Halushka PV, Rogers C, Whetsell A and Sagel
   J. Platelet adhesion and aggregation in diabetes mellitus. Metabolism. 28, 394-400, 1979.

6. Lagarde M, Bryon PA, Guichardant M and Dechavanne M. A simple method
   for platelet isolation from their plasma. Thrombos. Res. In press.

7. Born GVR. Aggregation of blood platelets by adenosine diphosphate
   and its reversal. Nature. 194, 927-929, 1962.

8. Lagarde M, Gharib A and Dechavanne M. A simple radiochemical assay
   of thromboxane B_2, 12-hydroxy-eicosatetraenoic acid (HETE) and 12-
   hydroxy-heptadecatrienoic acid (HHT) synthetized by human platelets.
   Clin. Chim. Acta 79, 255-259, 1977.

9. Lagarde M, Velardo B, Blanc M and Dechavanne M. Fatty acids bound
   to serum albumin decrease the half-life of thromboxane A_2.
   Submitted to publication.

10. Anderson MW, Crutchley DJ, Tainer BE and Eling TE. Kinetic studies
    on the conversion of prostaglandin endoperoxide PGH_2 by thromboxane
    synthase. Prostaglandins 16, 563-570, 1978.

11. Gorman RR, Bunting S and Miller OV. Modulation of human platelet
    adenylate cyclase by prostacyclin (PGX). Prostaglandins 13, 377-388,
    1977.

12. Gorman RR and Miller OV. Modulation of platelet cyclic nucleotide
    levels by PGE_1 and the prostaglandin endoperoxides PGG_2 and PGH_1.
    In : Prostaglandins in hematology. Silver MJ, Smith JB and Kocsis
    JJ (eds). New York. Spectrum Publications. 1977, 235-246.

13. Lapetina EG, Schmitges CJ, Chandrabose K and Cuatrecasas P. Cyclic
    AMP and prostacyclin inhibit platelet membrane phospholipase.
    Biochem. Biophys. Res. Commun. 76, 828-835, 1977.

13 THE STABILITY OF EICOSANOIDS: ANALYTICAL CONSEQUENCES

F.A. Fitzpatrick

Most experiments can be regarded as possible or impossible, and
sensible or senseless. The chemically unstable eicosanoids, such
as prostaglandin I_2 (PGI_2) and thromboxane A_2 (TxA_2) exist transiently.
Is it possible, or sensible, to measure these unstable agents, and
how do experimental conditions influence their measurements?

Bioassays (1), axiomatically, detect biologically active substances such as TxA_2 (2-3) and PGI_2 (4-5). However, bioassays require
meticulous attention to methodological details, and few bioassays are
quantitatively reliable (6). Assays that are more reliable and
effortless are preferable to bioassays, if the chemical nature of the
analyte permits their use.

PGI_2, commonly measured by bioassay, illustrates this. The
instability of PGI_2 originates in its vinyl ether functional group (7).
Vinyl ethers hydrolyze rapidly in aqueous solutions by an acid catalyzed process. Increasing alkalinity retards this hydrolysis. The
chemical nature of PGI_2 permits one to fix, temporarily, the hydrolysis of PGI_2 into 6-keto-$PGF_{1\alpha}$, by quenching a sample in alkali (pH
11-12) buffer at 0°C or lower. High performance liquid chromatography
in the reversed phase mode on a μBondapak® C18 column eluted with
acetonitrile/water, 20/80 v/v buffered at pH 9.3 with sodium borate
can then be used to separate intact PGI_2·Na from 6-keto-$PGF_{1\alpha}$ [Figure
1]. Under these chromatographic conditions there is no evident decomposition of PGI_2·Na during its transit through the column. For some
applications, detection and quantitation are based on ultraviolet
light absorption at 214 nanometers. The sensitivity of the technique
is 5-10 nanograms injected on-column (8). For applications requiring
greater sensitivity, the appropriate fraction can be collected; delib-
erately hydrolyzed, and subsequently measured as 6-keto-$PGF_{1\alpha}$ by
radioimmunoassay. The ability to stabilize PGI_2, chemically, and to
separate PGI_2 from 6-keto-$PGF_{1\alpha}$, chromatographically, forms a basis
for monitoring the ratio of PGI_2/6-keto-$PGF_{1\alpha}$ in many samples. It
is critical to avoid alcohols in the quenching or chromatographic
steps. PGI_2 and 6-keto-$PGF_{1\alpha}$, as hemi-ketals, can interact with

alcohols to form alkyl ketals. These products appear as distinct peaks during chromatography and complicate quantitation.

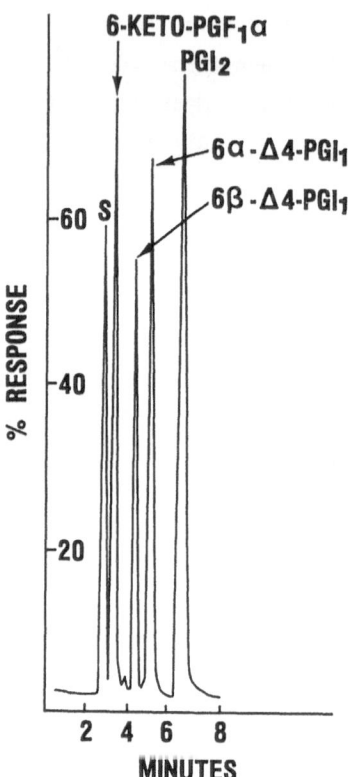

Figure 1. Typical Chromatogram of PGI$_2$Na and its decomposition product (6-keto-PGF$_{1\alpha}$) or contaminants (6α-, or 6β-Δ4-PGI$_1$)

Granstrom and Kindahl pioneered radioimmunoassay procedures to quanti-
tate both TxA_2, and TxB_2, its stable aqueous hydrolysis product
(9-10). Although described, originally, as an activity during bioassay
(2); and defined, structurally, by mass spectroscopy (3), the growth
in understanding the role of thromboxane A_2 has emerged from the
development and application of such sensitive, reliable radioimmunoassays (9-10). Some data derived from radioimmunoassays for TxB_2
illustrate how the actual experimental conditions can influence the
analysis.

Radioimmunoassay of TxB_2 formed during platelet aggregation, *in
vitro*, is common. The platelet system is a useful model because:
a) platelets are rich in cyclooxygenase and thromboxane synthetase
b) biochemical events (e.g. TxB_2 formation) can be correlated with
biological events (e.g. aggregation) c) platelets are plentiful
d) experiments are simple and advance the development of two fields
of research. Despite progress on the platelet-eicosanoid axis,
controversies about the most basic issues remain. Is TxA_2 necessary
for aggregation (11); or is it sufficient (12)? It is difficult to
reconcile data from different groups so the contradictions must be
real.

One source for the contradictions could be differences in
experimental conditions. Platelet experiments require either platelet
rich plasma (PRP), which is erythrocyte and lymphocyte depleted plasma
enriched in platelets by centrifugal separation; or washed platelets
suspended in a protein free balanced salt solution. To study the
platelet cyclooxygenase, directly, one adds arachidonic acid, exogenously, to either PRP or WP. The arachidonic acid is a substrate
for the cyclooxygenase enzyme, and its transformation product, PGH_2,
influences platelet function. To study the platelet thromboxane
synthetase, directly, one adds PGH_2 to PRP or WP. The PGH_2 is a
substrate for thromboxane synthetase, and its transformation product,
TxA_2 also, influences platelet function. There are other possible
aggregatory stimuli (e.g. collagen, thrombin, adenosine diphosphate,
epinephrine,) but arachidonic acid and PGH_2 affect the cyclooxygenase
and thromboxane synthetase with a minimal involvement of preceeding
enzymatic transformations. Typical experiments involve: a) preparation of PRP and/or washed platelet suspensions b) addition of arachidonic acid or PGH_2 c) measurement of aggregation d) measurement of
thromboxane B_2 and/or other products of intermediary metabolism in

platelets. Thromboxane B_2 radioimmunoassays, typically, involve:
a) sample withdrawal as a function of time b) sample transfer to
a medium that quenches the platelet cyclooxygenase or thromboxane synthetase c) dilution, if necessary, and RIA measurement.

Results show that arachidonic acid $[0-500 \ \mu g \text{-} ml^{-1}]$ causes a
dose-dependent aggregation of platelet rich plasma. The initiation
of aggregation; the rate of aggregation; and the maximal extent of
aggregation, all coincide with the rate of formation and accumulation
of TxB_2 measured by radioimmunoassay. The results are similar for
washed platelet suspensions aggregated with arachidonic acid; however,
washed platelets are sensitive to considerably lower concentrations
of arachidonic acid $(0 - 2.5 \ \mu g \text{-} ml^{-1})$. The results of such experiments
indicate that platelets transform arachidonic acid into PGH_2; then
the platelets transform PGH_2 into TxA_2, which hydrolyzes into TxB_2.
Radioimmunoassay determinations of TxB_2, evidently, reflect the
temporal and quantitative relationships between the thromboxane synthetase and platelet function.

Results are similar when one aggregates washed platelet suspensions with PGH_2. Exogenous addition of the immediate substrate for
the thromboxane synthetase bypasses the cyclooxygenase enzyme, but
TxB_2, measured by radioimmunoassay accumulates, and aggregation
accompanies the accumulation [Figure 2].

Of four possible experimental protocols: 1) washed platelets
plus arachidonic acid 2) washed platelets plus PGH_2 3) platelet rich
plasma plus arachidonic acid and 4) platelet rich plasma plus PGH_2,
only the first three give uniform results. The last protocol, platelet
rich plasma aggregated with PGH_2 is uncommon, and it produces uncon-
ventional results. Under experimental conditions otherwise identical
to the first three protocols, PGH_2 aggregates platelets in a conventional manner, but there is an apparent maximal production of TxB_2
prior to maximal aggregation, and the TxB_2 levels subsequently decrease
instead of accumulating as aggregation proceeds [Figure 3]. Control
experiments minimized the possibility that the TxB_2 radioimmunoassay
was inaccurate, or that it was responding to cross reacting material.
For example, the "burst" of measurable TxB_2 formation was substrate
(PGH_2) concentration dependent [Figure 4], and selective TxA_2
synthetase inhibitors blocked the formation of measurable TxB_2. The
disappearance, rather than accumulation, of measurable TxB_2 suggested

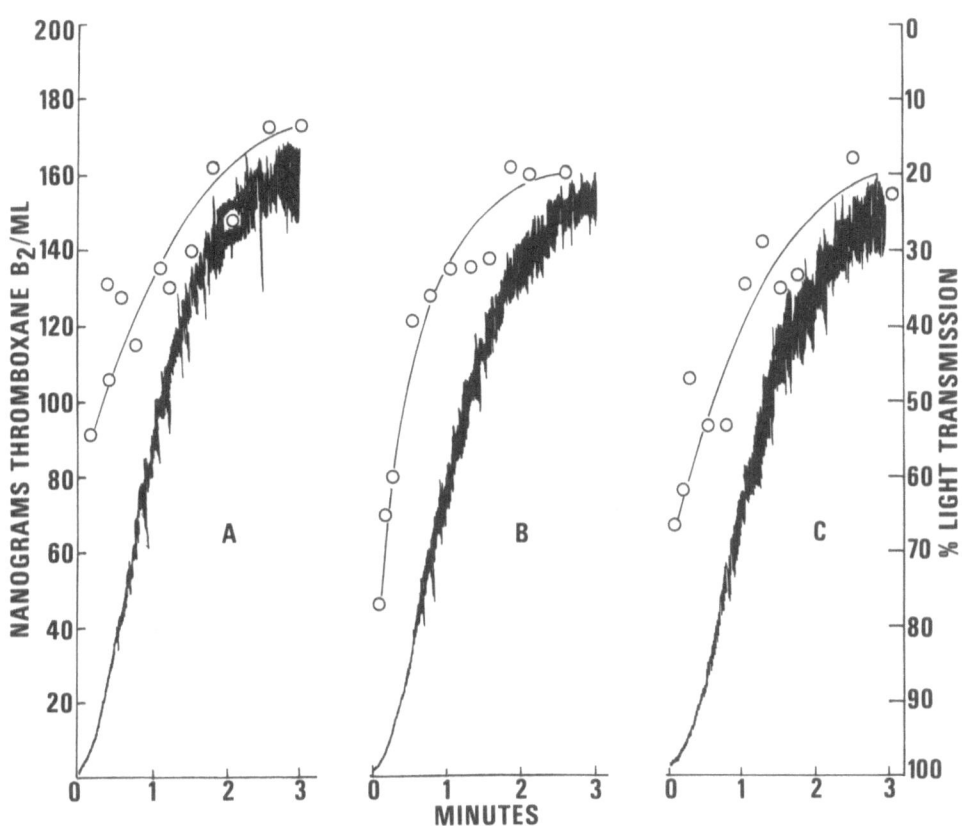

Figure 2. *Thromboxane B$_2$ formation (o-o-) during aggregation of washed platelets (1.0 ml, 10^9 platelets-ml^{-1}) with PGH$_2$ (1.0 μg). Results of three experiments.*

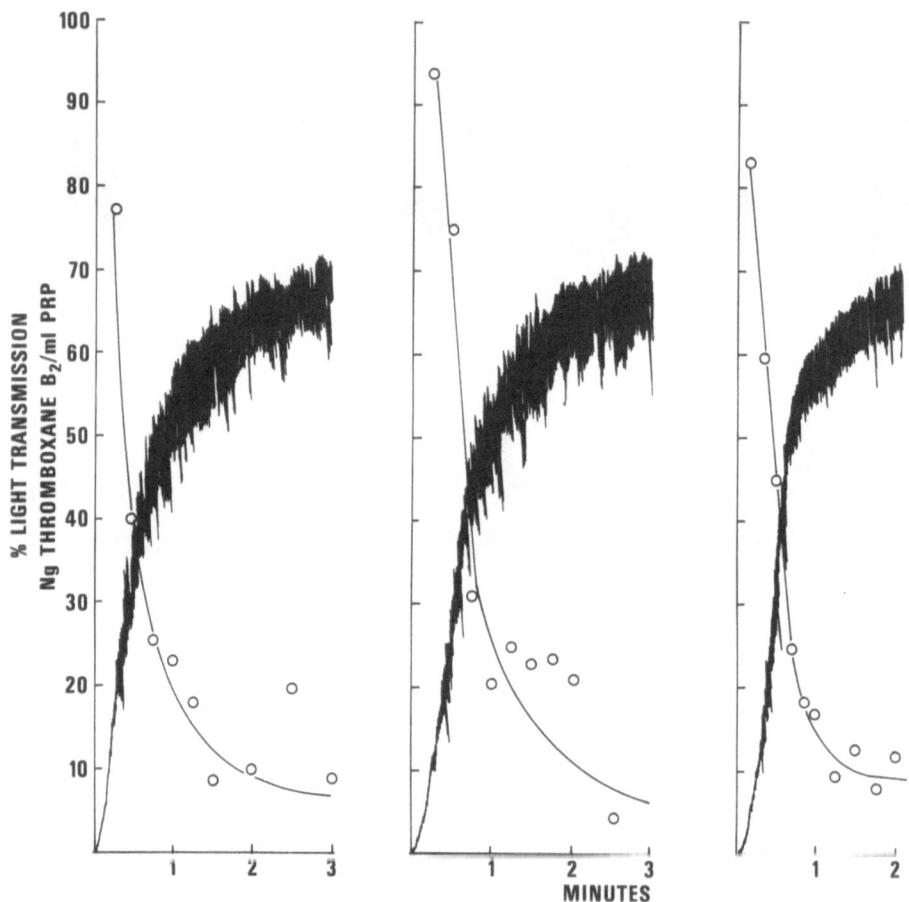

Figure 3. Thromboxane B₂ formation (-o-o-) during aggregation of platelet rich plasma (1.0 ml, 10⁹ platelets-ml⁻¹) with PGH₂ (1.0 μg). Results from four individual subjects. Compare with Figure 2.

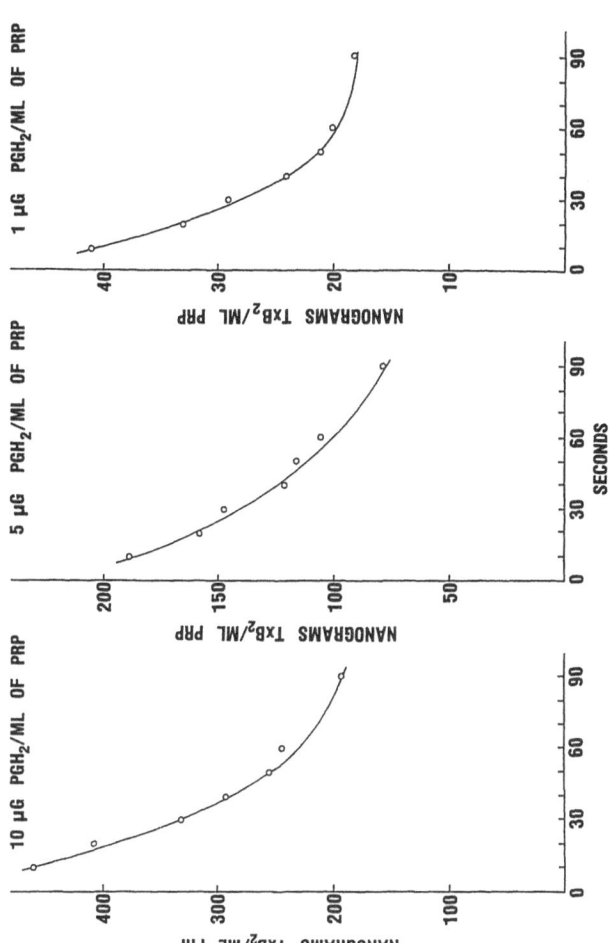

Figure 4. Platelet rich plasma transforms PGH_2 (1–10 µg PGH_2/ml PRP) into TxB_2 in a substrate dependent fashion.

that TxA_2 predominated in its labile form inside the aggregation cuvette, and the TxA_2 hydrolyzed to TxB_2, mainly, when it was transferred to the quenching solution. Evidence from experiments with different quenching solutions supported this interpretation. Samples (100 μl) quenched in acetone (100 μl), instead of citric acid, eliminated the "burst" of TxA_2 [Figure 5]. A plausible interpretation is that the labile epoxy bond of TxA_2 attached preferrentially to the protein precipitate, formed during acetone quenching, instead of hydrolyzing into TxB_2. Samples quenched in citric acid favor hydrolysis of TxA_2 into TxB_2 rather than preferential binding to protein. Experiments with $1-^{14}C-PGH_2$ substantiated the covalent binding of TxA_2 to plasma proteins. After aggregation, dialysis, and lyophilization, the protein residue quenched in acetone contained $30 \pm 4\%$ [n = 3 experiments] protein associated, non-dialyzable, radioactivity. There was no metabolic transformation of TxB_2 incubated (37°C) with platelet rich plasma for 60 minutes. When platelet rich plasma containing exogenously added TxB_2 was aggregated with ADP, the TxB_2 was recovered intact suggesting that platelet activation or aggregation is not accompanied by induction of TxA_2 or TxB_2 metabolizing systems.

The unusual profile of measurable TxB_2 formation and its relationship to the enzymology and biology of PGH_2 induced platelet aggregations leads to the conclusion that hydrolysis is not the exclusive fate of TxA_2 under some experimental conditions. This is illustrated by two hypothetical cases. In the first case, [Figure 6] we assume that TxA_2 disappears by hydrolysis only. If TxA_2 disappears by hydrolysis only, it is immaterial, analytically, if TxA_2 hydrolyzes within the PRP, inside an aggregometer cuvette, or within the quenching buffer, after its transfer from the aggregometer cuvette. The measurement for TxB_2 will reflect the composite level of TxA_2 plus TxB_2, regardless of their ratio. This model does not account for the data generated when exogenous PGH_2 aggregates PRP.

In the second case, [Figure 7] we assume that TxA_2 disappears by hydrolysis and covalent binding to proteins. In this case, a portion of the enzymatic capacity of the platelet thromboxane synthetase is masked, because the TxA_2 covalently bound to proteins is undetectable by assays that measure TxB_2. These assays measure the TxA_2 diverted to a "hydrolysis pool", but there is another "protein bound" pool that may be relevant clinically and diagnostically. This model accounts for the data generated when exogenous

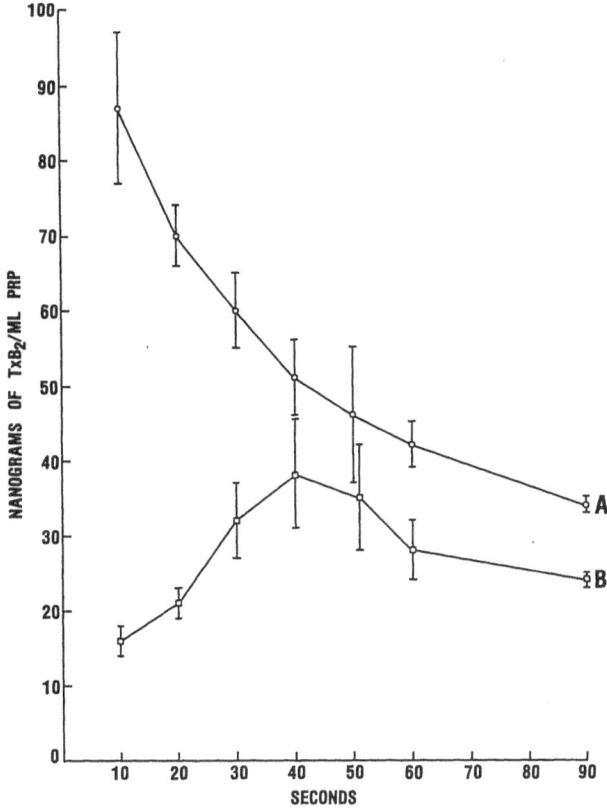

Figure 5. The pattern of measurable TxB$_2$ was altered when samples
from the aggregation of PRP (2.0 ml) with PGH$_2$ (4 µg)
were quenched in acetone (50 µl) [Trace B] compared to
identical samples quenched in 2M citric acid (0.01 ml)
[Trace A]. Values shown are the mean ± relative
standard deviations from 4 experiments quenched by each
technique. The disappearance of the initial "burst"
is consistent with TxA$_2$, in its labile form, binding
covalently to the protein precipitate.

WHAT IS THE FATE OF THROMBOXANE A_2 IN PLATELET RICH PLASMA?

CASE I: THROMBOXANE A_2 "DISAPPEARS" BY HYDROLYSIS ONLY

TIME	AMOUNT OF TxA$_2$ IN PRP	AMOUNT OF TxA$_2$ CONVERTED TO TxB$_2$ BY HYDRO-LYSIS WITHIN THE PRP DURING AGGREGATION	AMOUNT OF TxB$_2$ IN PRP AFTER ACID QUENCHING: MEASURABLE TxB2 FORMED BY FORCED HYDROLYSIS
0	0	0	0
1	20	0	20
2	100	0	100
3	80	20	100
4	60	40	100
5	40	60	100
6	20	80	100
7	0	100	100
8	0	100	100

Figure 6. An examination of projected TxB$_2$ levels for a hypothetical aggregation experiment (PRP + PGH$_2$) in which TxA$_2$ "disappears" by hydrolysis exclusively.

WHAT IS THE FATE OF THROMBOXANE A_2 IN PLATELET RICH PLASMA?

CASE II: THROMBOXANE A_2 "DISAPPEARS" BY <u>HYDROLYSIS</u> AND COVALENT BINDING TO PROTEINS

TIME	AMOUNT OF TxA₂ IN PRP	AMOUNT OF TxA₂ CONVERTED TO TxB₂ BY HYDROLYSIS WITHIN PRP DURING AGGREGATION	AMOUNT OF TxA₂ "MASKED" OR "REMOVED" BY CO-VALENT BINDING TO PROTEINS WITHIN THE PRP DURING AGGREGATION	AMOUNT OF MEASURABLE TxB₂: COMPOSITION OF PRP AFTER ACID QUENCH	
0	0	0	0	0	
1	20	0	0	20	
2	100	0	0	100	
3	80	10	10	90	10
4	60	20	20	80	20
5	40	30	30	70	30
6	20	40	40	60	40
7	0	50	50	50	50
8	0	50	50	50	50
9	0	50	50	50	50

Figure 7. An examination of projected TxB₂ levels for a hypo-thetical aggregation experiment (PRP + PGH₂) in which TxA₂ "disappears" by hydrolysis and covalent binding to plasma proteins.

PGH_2 aggregates PRP. Covalent binding represents an important alternative "fate" for labile eicosanoids. Identification and measurement of eicosanoids in the "protein bound" compartment represents a principal problem now facing researchers in this field.

References

1. Vane J: The use of isolated organs for detecting active substances in the circulating blood. Brit J Pharmacol Chemotherap 23: 360-378, 1964.

2. Vargaftig B, Zirinis J: Platelet aggregation induced by arachidonic acid is accompanied by release of potential inflammatory mediators distinct from PGE_2 and $PGF_{2\alpha}$. Nature New Biology 244: 114-116, 1973.

3. Hamberg M, Svensson J, Samuelsson B: Thromboxanes: a new group of biologically active compounds derived from prostaglandin endoperoxides. Proc Natl Acad Sci USA 72: 2994-2998, 1975.

4. Moncada S, Gryglewski R, Bunting S, Vane J: An enzyme isolated from arteries transforms prostaglandin endo- peroxides to an unstable substance that inhibits platelet aggregation. Nature 263: 663-665, 1976.

5. Pace-Asciak C, Wolfe L: Polyhydroxy cyclic ethers formed from tritiated arachidonic acid by acetone powders of sheep seminal vesicles. Biochemistry 10: 3664-3669, 1971.

6. Roth J, Lesniak M, Bar R, Muggeo M, Megyesi K, Harrison L, Flier J, Wachschlicht-Rodbard H, Gorden P: An introduction to receptors and receptor disorders. Proc Soc Exp Biol Med 162: 3-12, 1979.

7. Chiang Y, Kresge A, Cho M: Acid catalyzed hydrolysis of prostacyclin: origin of the unusual lability. J C S Chem Comm: 129-130, 1979.

8. Wynalda M, Fitzpatrick F: High performance liquid chromatographic assay for prostacyclin. J Chromatogr 176: 413-417, 1979.

9. Granstrom E, Kindahl H, Samuelsson B: Radioimmunoassay for thromboxane B_2. Anal Lett 9: 611-627, 1976.

10. Granstrom E, Kindahl H, Samuelsson B: A method for measuring the unstable thromboxane A_2: radioimmunoassay of the derived mono-o-methyl thromboxane B_2. Prostaglandins 12: 929-941, 1976.

11. Fitzpatrick F, Gorman R: Platelet rich plasma transforms exogenous prostaglandin H_2 into thromboxane A_2. Prostaglandins 14: 881-889, 1977.

12. Needleman P, Minkes M, Raz A: Thromboxanes: selective biosynthesis and distinct biological properties. Science 193: 163-165, 1976.